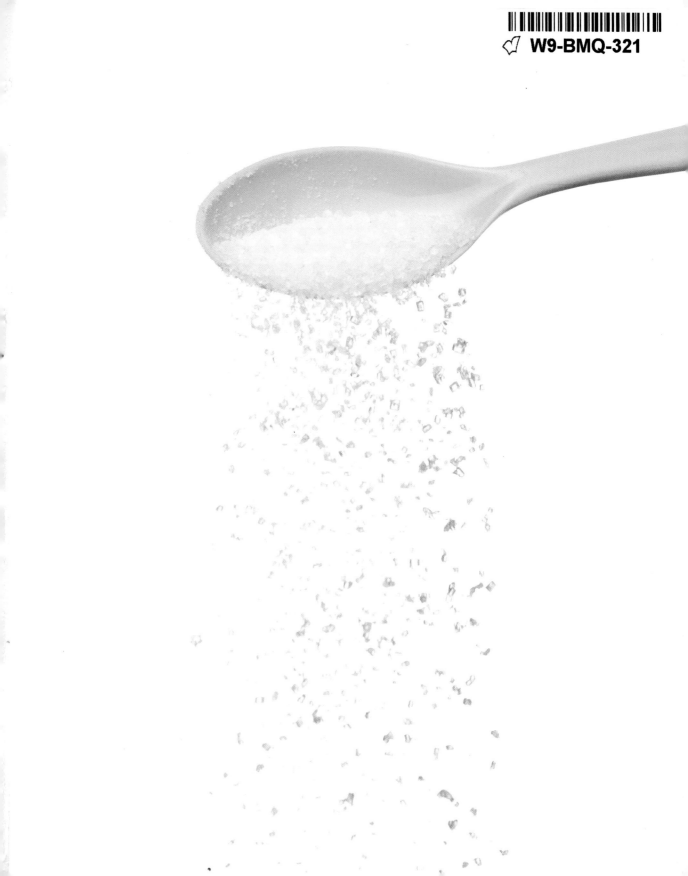

First published in 2013 by Victory Belt Publishing Inc.

ISBN-13: 978-1-936608-11-9

The information included in this book is for educational purposes only. It is not intended or implied to be a substitute for professional medical advice. The reader should always consult his or her healthcare provider to determine the appropriateness of the information for their own situation or if they have any questions regarding a medical condition or treatment plan. Reading the information in this book does not create a physician-patient relationship.

Victory Belt® is a registered trademark of Victory Belt Publishing Inc.

Book design: Joan Olkowski, Graphic D-signs, Inc.
Food photography: Diane Sanfilippo
Cover portrait: Kelli Beavers
Hair: Samantha Gaiser
Make-up: Hayley Mason

Printed in the USA

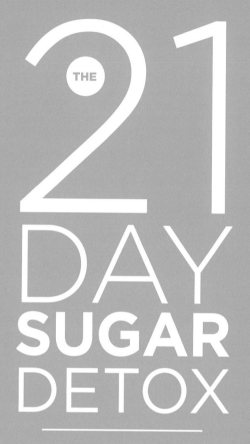

THE 21 DAY SUGAR DETOX

BUST SUGAR & CARB CRAVINGS NATURALLY

DIANE SANFILIPPO, BS, NC

VICTORY BELT PUBLISHING INC.
LAS VEGAS

TABLE OF CONTENTS

The 21-Day Sugar Detox

program **basics**

my sugar story

"I like to eat and the only thing I've ever been addicted to in my life is sugar." —Crispin Glover

I grew up in a small New Jersey town, around the corner from a 24-hour convenience store. It sold everything from 64-ounce sodas to magazines, emergency car parts, lottery tickets, and candy—*lots* of candy. The candy aisle became a bit of a home to me. If I earned $2 for completing some chores, you can bet that every penny of it was going to be spent on Snickers, Rolos, Three Musketeers, Blow Pops, Tootsie Rolls, and Jolly Ranchers.

You could say that I was The Candy Girl. If I had candy in my possession, I was going to eat it—any time of the day or night. On November 1 I'd wake up and have Halloween candy for breakfast. Sweets didn't stand a chance with me. My mom would try to hide them, but I knew all her hiding spots.

This relationship with sugar and sweets didn't end with my youth. Nope, it followed me well into adulthood, when I had free rein to eat whatever I wanted, whenever I wanted. Birthday cake for breakfast? Yes, please! Leftover pie for an afternoon snack? You better believe it.

It wasn't just sweets, either—I loved sugar in any form. I'm talking about refined carbs that turn to sugar in your body (which you'll learn about later), like bagels, pretzels, sandwich bread, and pasta. I was a high school athlete, so I figured I needed to carb up, right? Well, when I got to college, I kept eating like an athlete but stopped training like one—and I packed on the pounds. Thirty-five of them, to be exact.

When I finally realized that I had to do something about what had happened to my body, I dove headfirst into the point-counting, fat-fearing world of dieting and label reading. I checked the numbers (calories, fat, and fiber) on everything I ate—but I never read the ingredients. If it was a processed "health" food, I ate it: high-fiber cereal, soy cheese, low-fat granola bars, and non-fat anything. I'd eat meals that left me feeling full for maybe two hours and then reach for snacks to prop up my energy level and keep me from zombie-level hunger.

I was the friend in the group who got hangry (hungry + angry = hangry!) if we had to wait more than 20 minutes to be seated at a restaurant. I carried those popular low-fat granola bars in my purse—as if they were helping. They weren't. I knew I was on a blood sugar roller-coaster, but I didn't know how to get off it! I thought I was supposed to eat every two hours. "Eat small meals." "Eat some carbs to get your blood sugar up." That's what they say, isn't it?

Now, there's a difference between getting hungry as you naturally should, and getting to that hangry place because you've overdone it on bad carbs and your blood sugar is trying to make sense of things—jumping up only to come crashing back down. I never knew that it was possible to get hungry *without* also getting shaky, feeling like I was going to pass out, sweating, or even feeling nauseated, like I would do anything to get my hands on something to eat.

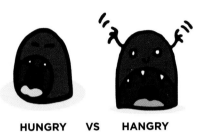

HUNGRY   VS   HANGRY

Fast-forward several years, and the weight had come off because I was undereating and over-exercising. I won't argue that there are lots of ways to lose weight, but my approach at that time wasn't a healthy one. I felt awful. My body wasn't getting the nourishment it needed from the low-calorie, low-fat, low-nutrition food I was eating! I was still on the blood sugar roller-coaster, chasing my energy around all day with food.

Eventually I learned from my personal trainer that eating meals that were more balanced—with adequate protein and plenty of fat, as well as veggies—could help me feel better. I resisted at first, because I was convinced that eating fat would make me fat. Boy, was I wrong. When I finally decided to stop being afraid of fat and give this new approach a shot, I ate a reasonably sized meal of chicken thighs and kale cooked in some coconut oil, and I wasn't hungry again for several hours. And when I got hungry, I just got hungry. I was finally able to eat a meal and feel satisfied.

What a difference protein and fat can make! Once I cut out the sugar and refined foods, eliminated gluten, and followed that up by cutting other grains and legumes, my blood sugar stabilized. It was like a miracle. I could go out with plans of being gone for over an hour and not have to jam a snack into my purse—food freedom!

After a year of gloriously even blood sugar levels, I had a slip-up. It was around four in the afternoon, and I was working at my local Starbucks, just a few blocks from my apartment. I had worked through lunch and was hungry—*really* hungry. I knew way better than to go so long without eating, but I had done it anyway. And then, instead of taking myself home to eat, I stopped at the candy store.

The Candy Girl had been dormant for many years, but she hadn't quite been obliterated yet! I probably bought a quarter pound of

WHAT IS GLUTEN?
The word *gluten* is often used as an umbrella term for the gliadin protein or a number of other constituents in grains to which people can react negatively. Gluten is found in grains and by-products of wheat, barley, rye, triticale, oats (typically from cross-contamination), and other grains, as well as in some other foods where these grains are used in processing. ●

gummy candies, licorice, and other assorted super-sugary goodies. And I ate the entire bag. At once.

About an hour later, I was in my apartment just beginning to cook dinner when it hit me. The after-effects of my massive sugar intake led to the hardest blood sugar crash I'd ever felt. I was right back to that full-blown hangry place—shaking, sweating, and feeling like I was going to pass out. I actually felt like I might fall to the floor. At the time, I was experimenting with raw milk in my diet, and luckily I had some in the fridge. I grabbed it and chugged a small glassful. And then another.

Once I finally started to feel better, I knew without a doubt that my dietary changes had been the right way to go—and I was never going to do that to my body again. Removing sugar and refined foods from my diet has given me the energy I always knew I should have, improved the quality of my sleep, and even helped to alleviate the chronic sinus infections I struggled with for many years. After years of consistently worsening dental health, I stopped developing cavities. To my surprise, my vision even improved, and an old contact lens prescription is now too strong. It's amazing what can happen when we give our bodies what they want, rather than simply what's readily available at every corner store.

As a result of my journey, my own blood sugar roller-coaster experiences, years of holistic nutritional studies, and then more years of working with clients as a nutrition consultant and teacher, I developed The 21-Day Sugar Detox. I wanted to give people a way to jump-start the process of kicking those sugar and carb cravings—and get them off the blood sugar roller-coaster.

The program has lived for several years as an eBook and thousands of people have successfully completed it, experiencing new things that they never thought possible just by kicking sugar to the curb.

My goal has been, and will continue to be, to show people how changing the balance of the food on their plates, as well as their habits around sweets and refined foods, will change their lives. I'm not here to discuss every medical and clinical issue that can arise as a result of sugar consumption; there are plenty of other books that do that. I'm here to guide you through this journey with an effective, clear-cut program that will liberate you from the chains of your cravings.

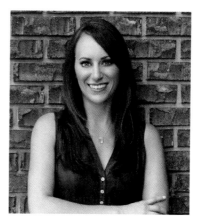

Yours in health,

Diane

introduction

"There are ways to cut cravings by naturally balancing your blood sugar." —Dr. Mark Hyman

Congratulations! You've already taken the first step in your journey to kicking your sugar addiction to the curb. I hope you've landed here because you already know—and likely feel—the negative effects that sugar has on your body.

If you're not entirely sure whether you need a sugar detox, take a moment to answer the following questions.

1. Do you crave sugar all day, every day—or even a few times a week? I'm talking about candy, sweets, chocolate, or lots of fruit.
2. Do you crave carbohydrates? These include bread, rice, pasta, pastries, cereal (yes, even oatmeal!), sandwiches, wraps, and breakfast bars.
3. Do you include something sweet with every meal or snack?
4. Do you experience spikes and dips in your energy levels throughout the day?
5. Do you often feel tired upon waking in the morning?
6. Do you drink alcoholic beverages daily or multiple times per week?
7. Are you trying to burn body fat?
8. Are you following a low-fat, whole-grain-rich diet that just isn't working?
9. Does the way you eat leave you feeling unsatisfied, hungry, and grazing on snacks every 2 to 3 hours?
10. Do you follow a clean-eating type of lifestyle (including, but not limited to, Paleo, primal, low-carb, vegetarian, Weston Price, and real food), but still experience carb or sugar cravings?

If you're like most people and answered yes to at least one of these questions, then you're a good candidate for this three-week program. Welcome! You're about to embark on a challenge that will be tough, but well worth it—I promise.

Sugar is a sneaky thing. It doesn't just cause cravings and make you fat; consuming too much of it can lead to all kinds of health issues, both in the short term and in the long term. To give you a bit more grounding here, let's look at a handful of less-obvious signs of sugar addiction, chronically erratic blood sugar levels, and nutrient deficiencies that may be caused by overconsumption of nutrient-poor carbohydrate foods:

SHORT TERM

Mood swings
Acne, rashes
Premenstrual
 syndrome (PMS),
 painful periods
Unrestful sleep
Fatigue

Muscle fatigue or
 weakness
Susceptibility to
 colds and flu
Other food
 addictions

LONG TERM

Anemia
Depression, anxiety
Cystic acne, ec-
 zema, psoriasis
PCOS, infertility
Insomnia
Adrenal fatigue or
 dysfunction

Myelopathy,
 neuropathy
Insulin resistance,
 type 2 diabetes
Alzheimer's disease
Substance abuse

JUST SAY NO TO GMO
By avoiding processed foods, you're also avoiding GMO ingredients, as 55% of the sugar in processed foods is genetically modified. The jury is still out on how genetically modified organisms (GMO) affect our health. I don't recommend risking it. ●

When I talk about being addicted to sugar, I'm not just talking about foods that you know to be sweet, or even candy itself. Unless you avoid packaged and processed foods entirely, you probably eat way more sugar than you think! The foods available in today's grocery stores are a veritable minefield, with added sugars hidden in nearly everything—breads, pasta sauces, salad dressings, "natural" peanut butter, "healthy" cereals, and even deli meats. These foods have been scientifically engineered to appeal to your senses at both a conscious and a subconscious level. Food scientists are constantly working on ways to strike just the right balance of sweet/salty/fatty, or at least the sensations of these tastes, to keep you coming back for more. Have you ever noticed that there's sodium in soda pop? So the very thing you're drinking to attempt to quench your thirst is actually going to make you even thirstier! Tricky, right? And that can of soda contains about 10 teaspoons of sugar, too. According to the Centers for Disease Control and Prevention, roughly 13% of adults' total daily caloric intake between 2005 and 2010 came from added sugars. That's about 22 teaspoons a day! When you avoid added sugars, you do yourself a favor by eliminating many packaged foods from your diet. In turn, you eliminate many other harmful ingredients and preservatives.

Even though it may feel like the deck is stacked against you, this book is here to help. With The 21-Day Sugar Detox, you can educate yourself about what you're eating and what those foods do to your body, and you can break the cycle of sugar addiction.

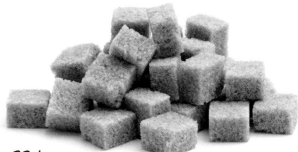
22 teaspoons of sugar

What is The 21-Day Sugar Detox?

The 21-Day Sugar Detox (21DSD) is a real food-based program designed to reduce and/or eliminate your cravings for sugar and carbohydrates. Through this three-week program, which focuses on quality protein, healthy fats, and good carbs, you'll change not only the foods you eat, but also your habits around food, and even the way your palate reacts to different foods. Removing added sugars and very sweet foods retrains your taste buds to perceive sweetness, and you'll find that foods you once thought weren't sweet at all become quite sweet as the days pass. Even the treat recipes in this book will taste quite different to you on Day 21 than they do on Day 1!

The 21DSD is not a no-carb or even a very low-carb eating plan. You will eat plenty of carbohydrates, including unlimited amounts of crunchy and leafy vegetables, as well as limited fruits and even some slightly starchier vegetables like beets and pumpkin. You'll just be eating *good* carbs—not the bad kinds that drain your energy and make losing body fat an uphill battle.

What you'll experience on this program will be different from a lot of other "diet" programs out there. By changing the foods you eat every day, you will begin to gain a new understanding of how food works in your body—and just how much nutrition affects your entire life.

Beyond helping you bust sugar and carb cravings, this program should serve as a real nutritional jump-start. You'll likely complete The 21DSD and continue eating this way much of the time thereafter because you'll feel so amazing. You may notice changes that you didn't expect, such as increased energy, better focus, and deeper, more restful sleep—along with some that you probably do expect, such as freedom from cravings and from needing the comfort of sugar at stressful times.

In the following pages, I'll explain lots of reasons why avoiding sugar in many forms is a good idea, but ultimately it's not my aim to convince you that you need to change your relationship with sugar. That's what this three-week program, and the revelations you'll experience once you are finished, will do for you!

HEALTHY FATS

You may be surprised by the fats that you should be eating for optimal health, including while on The 21DSD. They include naturally occurring saturated and monounsaturated fats like coconut oil, butter, lard, and olive oil. Eating these fats can help your body burn fat when you are no longer eating sugar! ●

What does it mean to detox from sugar?

Some of the most amazing things that happen in your life every day are the functions that your body carries out without any conscious effort from you. The autonomic, or involuntary, nervous system performs countless actions that control things like heartbeat, core body temperature, and even digestion. It also controls the functions of your organs, including detoxification.

De•tox (dee-toks) The process, real or perceived, of removing toxins from the body.

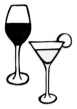

Luckily, you don't have to think about when or how to motivate your body to remove toxins from your system; your liver is designed to handle this job quite well. But what happens when you overload the liver with environmental toxins like smog or harsh chemical cleaners? Or alcohol, which needs to be cleared from your system before the liver can prioritize clearing other toxins? Or even sugar, which the liver has to work extra hard to clear when the bloodstream becomes overloaded with it?

When people think about a "detox," they're often thinking of a program that supports the liver with some kind of quick-fix or a bunch of supplements. But what about removing some of the everyday burden from the liver by eliminating alcohol and changing what kind of food enters your body? These simple changes can profoundly affect your body's ability to detoxify, enabling your liver to give priority to environmental toxins rather than focus on the insults from foods and drinks you consume. When you give your liver a break from alcohol and sugar, its newfound capacity to remove toxins from your body is one reason that some people who complete The 21-Day Sugar Detox experience headaches or fatigue for a couple of days early in the program.

But a second and often even more compelling aspect of a detox also needs to be recognized: the removal of toxic substances not just from your body, but also from your life. I'm talking about the habitual element of a detox, when you change what you do every day to eliminate those problematic substances.

Research supports the notion that it takes 21 days to form new habits, but the real-life implications of three weeks of making different choices and simply living differently are proof enough for most people. The research focuses mainly on the fact that the brain is extremely sensitive to—and tends to favor—repetition. The brain imprints the patterns of things you do and choices you make as habits, which makes it easier and easier to practice those habits again and again. Activities that become habits become more desirable to perform because they require less concentration. How is it that you get into your car and drive to work without a second thought? The route became habit at some point, after you took it a number of times. Once you dive in and give creating a new habit a shot, you may find that it's smooth sailing after even 14 days and that getting to Day 21 is a breeze.

While it isn't a direct "detox" effect, the way your tastes begin to change over the three weeks of this program will play a major role in supporting the new habits you form. The fruit that is included in the program is some of the least sweet-tasting

DETOX EFFECTS
When the liver is relieved of the burden of detoxifying alcohol and excess sugar, it can focus on working to release other toxic substances from the body's fat stores. This often leads to short-term discomfort such as headaches, joint or muscle pain, fatigue, changes in digestion, skin rashes, and decreased appetite. ●

available, and for good reason. I mentioned earlier that The 21DSD will change the way your palate reacts to foods. One of the issues that many people don't consider when attempting to beat sugar and carb cravings is that of sweet taste—almost regardless of its source. Some programs move you to artificial sweeteners as a replacement, but that's absolutely not going to happen on this program. Artificial sweeteners have no place in your everyday diet, whether you are on a sugar detox or not. The litany of negative effects of synthetic sweeteners, as well as the way the majority of them are produced, are reason enough for me to recommend against them. The way all sweeteners—caloric and non-caloric—can affect your tastes and the resulting physical and emotional reactions mean that they all need to be eliminated for your sugar detox to be effective.

There are many different takes on the concept of a detox. Most programs promote extremely restricted eating, such as eliminating all animal foods. Some encourage you to consume only shakes, juices, or smoothies for the duration of the program. Others rely heavily on supplements and very-low-calorie or very-low-fat diets to ensure success. The goal of any detox program should be to support your body in naturally cleansing itself of substances that create negative health effects.

To detox from sugar means not only to rid your body of cravings for it, but also to rid your daily life of the structure built around being a slave to when you eat sugar, how much you eat, and the form in which you eat it. Liberation from the physical desire for sugar, and the freedom to move through your days, weeks, months, or even years without feeling like you want or need to eat sugar—that's the goal of The 21-Day Sugar Detox.

artificial sweeteners

Artificial sweeteners have been identified as contributors to a litany of health problems, including but not limited to:

- migraines and headaches
- dizziness/poor equilibrium
- convulsions and seizures
- nausea and vomiting
- diarrhea

- fatigue and weakness
- changes in mood
- changes in vision
- changes in heart rate
- joint pain

- memory loss
- sleep problems/insomnia
- hives/rash
- weight-loss resistance

I don't know about you, but if I were suffering from any of these symptoms, the first thing I'd do to make my life easier would be to kick artificial sweeteners to the curb. For more on the far-reaching effects of these harmful products, I recommend checking out the articles on dorway.com and mercola.com. ●

Many people who are participating in The 21DSD find it helpful to have a network of support from others struggling with sugar cravings and sugar's negative effects and enjoy connecting with them via online forums, Facebook, or other social media outlets. Interacting with others while completing this program is not required, but it's strongly recommended! For a plethora of online resources, visit balancedbites.com/21DSD. ●

Is this the right program for you?

The 21-Day Sugar Detox is a fantastic program for a variety of personalities. It offers both a highly structured approach and a ton of flexibility within its scope. If you enjoy being told exactly what, when, and how much to eat each day, then following one of the 21-day meal plans will work perfectly for you. If you like to be creative and have flexibility with your meal planning, you can simply follow the Yes/No Foods List for your level while you build meals and snacks that fit within the program's guidelines.

If you're ready to commit to yourself, to choose foods that will help your body and support your goals, and to feel better, then this is the program for you.

If you know deep down that eating real, whole foods is the way to go, then this is the program for you.

If you're ready to get into the kitchen to make simple, delicious meals for yourself, then this is the program for you.

If you're looking for easy-to-understand descriptions of the negative effects of sugar that won't paralyze you with fear about choosing anything to eat, then this is the program for you.

If you don't need someone to beat you over the head with page after page of all the things you've been doing wrong for the last ten, twenty, thirty, or more years to convince you that you need to kick the sugar habit, then this is the program for you.

If you know that the answer to your cravings isn't a magic pill, potion, shake, or simply a handful of supplements that will miraculously take away your sugar cravings, then this is the program for you.

If you are, in fact, in the right place and this is the book and program for you, then let's move onward!

In this book, you'll find fantastic tools, tips, and resources to help you through the three weeks you'll spend ridding your body of sugar and carb cravings. First we'll look at the basic science of sugar and how your body processes carbohydrates. Then,

?

WHO SHOULDN'T DETOX?

If you are currently training for a marathon or other similar endurance-based competition, it would be best to wait until after the race to complete The 21DSD. ●

I'll walk you through how to prepare and what to expect on the program day-by-day. Throughout the book you'll find useful guides on topics like finding hidden sugar, which fats to eat and which to avoid, and even dining out 21DSD-style that you can refer to again and again—or grab them from my website (balancedbites.com/21DSD) and print copies to hang on your refrigerator for easy reference. You'll also learn where to find support beyond this book along your journey, and you'll get some tips and tricks for navigating life after you complete your detox.

Once you've read through the background information on the program, you'll take a short quiz to determine which level is right for you. The quiz will also point you to modifications to that level if appropriate (for example, you are pregnant or nursing, or you are an athlete). Each level includes a notes section to help you understand how your level differs from the other two, a Yes/No Foods List that outlines what to eat and avoid on that level, a 21-day meal plan using recipes from the book, and information about how to modify the program for your specific needs, if necessary. The delicious, easy recipes—a sampling of everything from breakfasts and main dishes to snacks and treats—round out the book. You can use them as you like within the structure of your selected level/modifications, or you can follow along exactly as your 21-day meal plan outlines—that part is entirely up to you!

I know what you're thinking: "This isn't going to be as easy as I thought!" Have no fear! In your hands you hold a fantastic resource based on my years of experience working with clients just like you—and thousands of program participants who have come before you. They've done it, and so can you. I'm here to help, every step of the way.

GET ONLINE

Visit my website at **balancedbites.com/21DSD** for all of the additional resources that accompany this book. ●

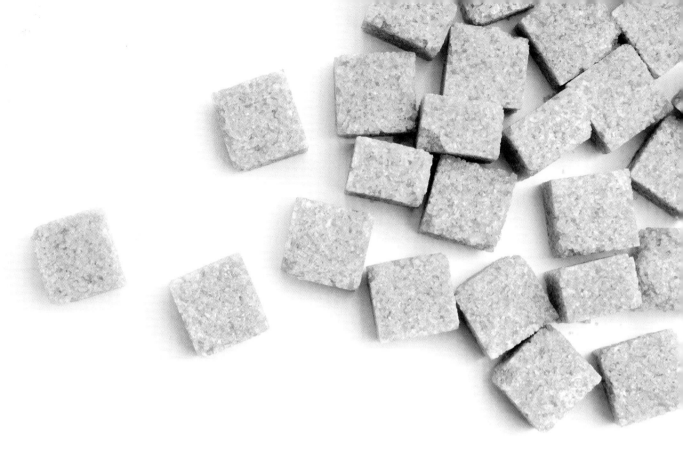

the science of sugar, simplified

"If it's popped, puffed, flaked, floured, shredded, or instant, it's been refined." —Radhia Gleis, PhD, MEd, CCN

Why do we crave sugar?

Before I walk you through how to best prepare for your 21DSD, let's get into some of the reasons why this program is going to improve your health from the inside out. Knowing what happens inside your body when you eat sugar and carbs—the science behind the cravings, sugar crashes, and other ill effects—should be a great source of motivation. Instead of just telling you not to eat a lot of sugar, I'm going to show you why it's a bad idea.

Long ago, the only sweet-tasting foods available were fruits and honey. Those foods were nutrient dense and were available only seasonally or where climates remained warm year-round. Naturally occurring sweet foods did not overstimulate the palate or lead to cravings as today's refined sweet foods do. Our ancestors consumed far fewer calories in the form of sugar than people do in our modern refined-sugar-and-carb landscape. Added sugars just didn't exist back then; only sweet natural foods did.

So why are we wired to love and seek out sweet foods? If sugar is bad for us, then why do we want to eat sweet things?

One word: dopamine.

Dopamine is a neurotransmitter (a chemical messenger that delivers signals to and from the brain) that helps control feelings of reward and pleasure. It is released for many healthy reasons, including physical touch and exercise. Dopamine is also released in response to the consumption of certain substances, including caffeine, narcotics, and sugar.

The dopamine response you get from eating sugar sends signals throughout your body that encourage you to continue to seek that pleasurable feeling. Now, this wouldn't be an inherently bad thing if the sugar you were eating every time you experienced this pleasure was nutrient dense, like some berries, and you were eating it in

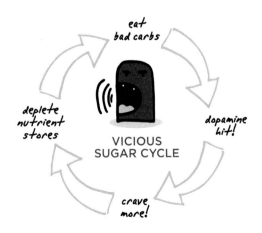

eat
bad carbs

deplete
nutrient
stores

dopamine
hit!

VICIOUS
SUGAR CYCLE

crave
more!

the overall context of a healthy and balanced diet. If you received this pleasure only from eating sugar where it naturally occurs, in fruit or honey, you would likely receive enough nutrition from the foods that stimulate this pleasure to calm the desire for more. In other words, you'd feel the pleasure from the sweet taste, but you wouldn't be hit with a subsequent craving. What happens today, however, isn't so straightforward. Not only do modern, refined forms of sugar trigger this release of dopamine, but they also rob your nutrient stores (more on this in a moment)—which leaves you with the constant desire for more sugar.

What makes up the foods you eat

For much of your life, you probably didn't think about what made up the food you were eating. It was just breakfast, lunch, and dinner—and maybe a snack or dessert in there as well. But knowing the makeup of foods goes a long way toward helping you determine whether they should earn their rightful place on your plate.

Let's start with some simple definitions of key nutrition terms:

Macronutrients are the calorie-carrying components that make up the foods you eat. Protein, carbohydrates, and fat are the three macronutrients. Protein and carbohydrates each carry 4 calories per gram, while fat carries 9 calories per gram.

A *calorie* is simply a unit of measurement that indicates how much energy you can expect to derive from the macronutrients that make up the food you are eating.

Micronutrients are non-calorie-carrying components that are found in foods: vitamins, minerals, trace minerals, organic acids, and phytochemicals. Micronutrients nourish your cells and enable them to create energy and metabolize consumed *macro*nutrients with ease.

Nutrient density refers to the quantity and variety of micronutrients carried by each calorie of a particular food. Note that when I talk about nutrient density, I'm not talking about foods that have been refined and then enriched or fortified. Those foods have been stripped of naturally occurring vitamins and minerals, and synthetic forms have been added back in the refining process.

• ENRICHED OR FORTIFIED •
What's the difference?

Enriched foods have had nutrients added back that are lost in processing. This is common with breads and other grain-based products.

Fortified foods have had nutrients added to them, regardless of whether they were there before processing. A great example is the recent boom in the addition of omega-3 fatty acids to foods like cereals and yogurt. ●

LEARN MORE
If you are interested in finding the foods that are the richest in nutrients, check out the book *Rich Food, Poor Food* by Dr. Jayson Calton and Mira Calton. ●

Good carbs, bad carbs

Now let's take a closer look at carbohydrates, the macronutrient you're taking in when you consume sugar. There is a lot of confusion about carbohydrates in the world of health and nutrition today. Which are good, and which are bad? Before I can explain the effects that good carbs and bad carbs have on your body, I need you to understand the difference between the two.

There are indeed good carbs and bad carbs. But I'm not talking about complex carbs versus simple carbs—like whole-grain bread versus white bread. You know, the story about how eating lots of whole-wheat bread is perfectly healthy, but white bread, well, that stuff's killing you? I am not like most other nutritionists out there who suggest that you can eat copious amounts of any foods you like, as long as the labels read "whole grain." You've heard that story before, and it hasn't helped—you're here, right? Let's look at this whole thing differently and examine the way your body really understands the distinction between good and bad carbs.

Good carbs come from whole, natural foods that are nutrient dense. Some good carbs that you'll be eating on The 21-Day Sugar Detox include broccoli, cauliflower, butternut squash, green apples, and carrots. Easy, right?

Bad carbs are a lot more complicated. First and foremost, bad carbs come from foods that are refined and man-made. How can you easily identify refined carbs, you ask? One of my favorite quotes on the subject is from nutritionist Radhia Gleis: "If it's popped, puffed, flaked, floured, shredded, or instant, it's been refined." This is a perfect way to wrap your head around all the refined foods that exist. Those whole-grain breads and pastas you've been so in love with, and that high-fiber flaked cereal made from seven different whole grains that are supposedly on a mission to make you healthier—well, they're all refined.

Bad carbs are macronutrient- and calorie-rich, but micronutrient-poor. You can eat tons of calories in bad carbs but never actually nourish your body with what it is looking for to be satisfied—vitamins and minerals!

Let's make this topic a bit clearer by comparing equal-calorie servings of sweet potato and bread made from unenriched wheat flour.

103 cals of sweet potato:
24 grams of carbohydrate
4 grams of dietary fiber
438% of the RDA for vitamin A
37% of the RDA for vitamin C
4% of the RDA for calcium
4% of the RDA for iron

101 cals of unenriched wheat bread:
20 grams of carbohydrate
1 gram of dietary fiber
0% of the RDA for vitamin A
0% of the RDA for vitamin C
0% of the RDA for calcium
1% of the RDA for iron

RDA = recommended daily allowance as set by the USDA

You can see that, in almost exactly the same number of calories, sweet potato packs a much more powerful nutrient punch than bread made from unenriched wheat flour.

Now, you will find breads, cereals, and other refined foods that claim to have high levels of vitamins and minerals. These enriched and fortified foods may look great on paper, but added synthetic nutrients can't compare to naturally occurring ones. Refined breads and cereals are sprayed with synthetic vitamins and minerals and sold to you as nutrient-dense foods. But you're smarter than that—and so is your body. What's so powerful about eating unrefined, unfortified whole-foods is that the nutrients are natural and synergistically balanced—in a way your body can use with ease and efficiency. When nutrients are added to foods in synthetic forms and without their co-factors (the complementary nutrients that are needed for proper absorption and utilization), your body simply cannot use them appropriately. For example, adding calcium to a breakfast cereal doesn't mean your body will properly absorb and utilize the extra calcium. However, when calcium is naturally present in whole foods that also contain the co-factors of vitamins A, D, K2, and magnesium, it can be absorbed by the body and used to strengthen bones.

always read ingredients

Food manufacturers rely on the fact that most people are going to read the Nutrition Facts portion of a label and never gaze down at the long list of lab-created ingredients that you can't pronounce. Below you'll see some ingredient lists from popular "health" foods sold today; it may be quite eye-opening to you! In **bold** you'll notice natural or naturally derived sweeteners, and in ***bold italics*** you'll see artificial sweeteners. Note that ingredients are listed in order of how much of each item is included in the product. Food manufacturers often use multiple sweeteners to attempt to hide the fact that there may be more sweetener in the product than almost anything else!

Kashi GOLEAN Crunch! Cereal
Ingredients: Kashi Seven Whole Grains & Sesame Blend (Whole Hard Red Wheat, Brown Rice, Barley, Triticale, Oats, Rye, Buckwheat, Sesame Seeds), Soy Flakes, **Brown Rice Syrup**, **Dried Cane Syrup**, Chicory Root Fiber, Whole Grain Oats, Expeller Pressed Canola Oil, **Honey**, Salt, Cinnamon, Mixed Tocopherols for Freshness.

Yoplait Light Strawberry yogurt
Ingredients: Cultured Pasteurized Grade A Nonfat Milk, Strawberries, Modified Corn Starch, **Sugar**, Kosher Gelatin, Citric Acid, Tricalcium Phosphate, ***Aspartame***, Potassium Sorbate Added to Maintain Freshness, ***Acesulfame Potassium***, Natural Flavor, Red #40, Vitamin A Acetate, Vitamin D3.

Wheat Thins Original crackers
Ingredients: Whole Grain Wheat Flour, Unbleached Enriched Flour (Wheat Flour, Niacin, Reduced Iron, Thiamine Mononitrate {Vitamin B1}, Riboflavin {Vitamin B2}, Folic Acid), Soybean Oil, **Sugar**, Cornstarch, **Malt Syrup (From Barley and Corn)**, Salt, **Invert Sugar**, Leavening (Calcium Phosphate and/or Baking Soda), Vegetable Color (Annatto Extract, Turmeric Oleoresin). BHT Added to Packaging Material to Preserve Freshness.

eating fat on The 21-Day Sugar Detox

While on The 21-Day Sugar Detox, you will build meals and snacks that are focused on the right kinds of carbohydrates as well as quality protein and fat sources. Since you will likely reduce your overall carbohydrate intake, you're going to have to eat more of something else to balance out your plate. What's that going to be? That's easy—fat.

Fat serves as a perfect, long-lasting fuel source for your body, but here's the catch: Your body can't efficiently burn fat for fuel (from your food or from your fanny) if you are eat-ing a steady stream of lots of carbohydrates. In order to become what is called "fat-adapted," meaning that your body knows how to effectively use fat for fuel, you have to stop giving it carbs all day, every day. And this is great news because it means that you don't have to eat every couple of hours to "fuel your metabolism." Quite the contrary! When you stop feeding yourself so many carbs and stop fearing natural, healthy fats (see page 61 because this may not mean what you think), your body relearns how to make it through the day. It burns not only the fat you eat, but also the extra "food" you have stored as body fat—the same fat you've been trying to burn off by cranking away on the elliptical machine for years.

I know what you're think-ing: "But how does that work? I thought I was sup-posed to eat lots of healthy whole grains and plenty of fruit to keep myself in shape!" Well, the answer is all about hormones and how they respond to the food you eat, which we will get to in just a moment.

Why is nutrient density so important?

Whole, unrefined, nutrient-dense sources of carbohydrates like vegetables, fruits, roots, and tubers give your body everything it needs to effectively turn the calories in those foods into energy, right in one package. In other words, eating whole, nutrient-dense foods enables you to make nutritional deposits into your body's "energy bank account." Nutrient-poor foods like sugar, on the other hand, ask your body for a withdrawal without making a deposit in return.

Let me explain what that means. To metabolize carbohydrates and turn them into energy, your body needs to use micronutrients—in particular, B vitamins and the minerals phosphorus, magnesium, iron, copper, manganese, zinc, and chromium. Bad carbs don't contain those vitamins and minerals in naturally occurring forms. Without both macronutrients *and* micronutrients in your food, your energy levels would plummet because your cells literally wouldn't be able to make energy and power your body. And they likely *do* plummet if you're eating lots of bad carbs all the time!

THERE'S SUGAR IN THAT?!
Some products on grocery store shelves that you may be shocked to see contain added sugars include ketchup, salad dressings, tomato/pasta sauces, crackers, dried fruits (aren't they sweet enough al-ready?!), deli meats, sausages, and "natural" nut butters. ●

Low nutrient density explains why a diet rich in bad carbs leaves you feeling tired and often depleted of energy. It's also why you feel the need to eat more and more—because your body is telling you to eat more food to get nutrients in! Except it doesn't want you to eat more of the bad stuff; it's begging you to eat good stuff loaded with vitamins and minerals to satisfy that need for micronutrients at the cellular level. The problem is, what's usually most readily available isn't the good stuff—unless you plan ahead! You'll learn just how critical planning and preparing are to your success on The 21-Day Sugar Detox on page 32.

Let's look at another real-life example of two foods, a good carb and a bad carb, and see how this scenario plays out.

Just 4 teaspoons of white table sugar (a bad carb) delivers about 60 calories in carbohydrate form. That's it. It doesn't give you anything else—no nutrients at all. You've heard the term *empty calories*, right? This is exactly what it means.

On the other hand, 1 cup of chopped cooked broccoli (a good carb) contains about 60 calories in carbohydrate form, but it also gives you B vitamins, phosphorus, magnesium, iron, copper, manganese, zinc, and chromium—the exact micronutrients your body needs to metabolize those carbohydrates. (It also gives you tons of vitamin C and vitamin K1 as well as vitamin E, folate, potassium, beta-carotene, calcium, zinc, and selenium.) As a result, your cells receive all of what they need from the broccoli you've eaten—and you're satisfied, not reaching for more and more carbs!

Choosing which carbohydrate foods to eat while on The 21-Day Sugar Detox will be quite simple: You're going to eat all good carbs and no bad ones. I provide easy Yes/No Foods Lists for each level of the program, as well as modifications for those of you who may need to tweak things—for instance, if you need extra energy for intense exercise, if you're pregnant or nursing, or if you eat a pescetarian diet.

How your body breaks down carbs

Now that you know the difference between good carbs and bad carbs, I'll explain what happens inside your body when you eat carbs. For this basic breakdown, I'm going to talk about all carbohydrates. Anything you eat that is not protein or fat is a carbohydrate—from bread, pasta, rice, and candy to broccoli, butternut squash, berries, and basil. Now, it's true that there are trace amounts of protein and fat in those foods, but the major macronutrient they represent is carbohydrate.

When you eat carbohydrate foods, your body gets to work breaking them down into a usable form of energy called *glucose* (a simple sugar), as well as vitamins and minerals. A sweet potato isn't a useful source of energy until your digestive system

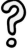

GOT MICRONUTRIENTS?
Common symptoms of micronutrient deficiencies that can be remedied by replacing bad carbs with good carbs include headaches, fatigue, bleeding gums, bruising easily, joint or limb pain, and anemia. ●

has taken it apart. As you eat that sweet potato, your digestive system releases enzymes that break it down into smaller "pieces."

Imagine that you just bought a brand-new box of Legos. Inside the box are a bunch of colored bricks, all connected to one another sort of haphazardly. But in order to build something out of those bricks, or even to put them away in the color-coded storage bins you have in your closet, you have to separate them into single pieces first. Likewise, your body needs to break down carbohydrate into glucose before it can be used or stored.

How glucose gets stored: insulin at work

Imagine that once you open that box of Legos, you can hold only a few blocks in your hand; the rest must either go into the storage bins or be used to build something. Similarly, you can't keep more than 4 grams of glucose in your bloodstream at any given time; it needs to be either used or stored.

Insulin is a storage hormone released by your pancreas in response to carbohydrates in your diet (a bit is released in response to protein as well). Its job is to send a message to your cells to let nutrients (including glucose)

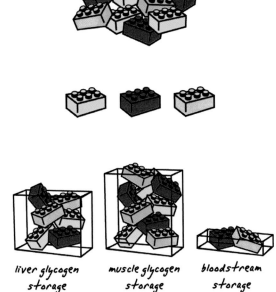

liver glycogen storage

muscle glycogen storage

bloodstream storage

in. When you eat carbohydrates, your body efficiently gets to work to release insulin and put the resulting glucose in your body's "storage bins": your liver and your muscles. Glucose that is put into those storage bins is called *glycogen*.

Now, there are tissues in your body that need small amounts of glucose to be replenished when your body's stores are low: your brain and your red blood cells. Before glucose gets stored in your liver and muscles, your liver, which is the master regulator of blood glucose levels, runs a check to make sure that your brain and red blood cells get what they need. Then it can move on to storing what's left of that glucose.

As you eat more and more carbohydrates, your body responds with more and more insulin to help store that glucose for later use. There's a catch, though: Just as your Lego storage bins can hold only so many Legos, your body has limited storage space for carbohydrates. The exact amount of carbohydrate that the body can store as glycogen in the liver and muscles varies from person to person.

So what happens when your body's carbohydrate "storage bins" are full? If you kept buying new Legos without ever taking the pieces you already owned out of the bins to build new creations, the bins would overflow, and you would have a big mess. Well, in your body, the carbohydrates you eat that your body doesn't use up for activity/exercise and doesn't have room to store as glycogen are converted to fat! While the body has limited storage for carbohydrates, it has unlimited storage for fat—sneaky, right? This fat is in the form of either 1) triglycerides, which are circulating blood fats, or 2) adipose, which is body fat.

Some basic carbohydrate math

To sum it up, your total carbohydrate storage capacity = liver storage + muscle storage + carbohydrates you burn in a day (that's your resting metabolic rate plus any carbs you burn with activity or exercise).

If carbohydrates eaten > liver storage + muscle storage + carbohydrates you burn in a day, then your body has no choice but to store the excess as fat. How and where you store your extra fat is determined largely by genetic predisposition.

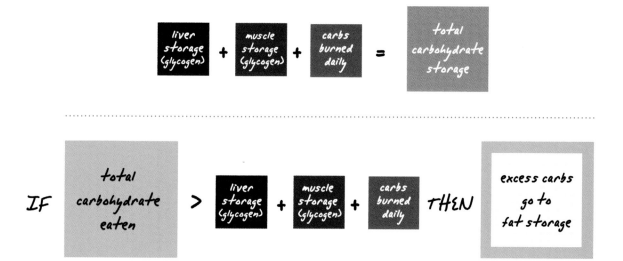

So how do you make sure that your body isn't getting more carbohydrates than it needs and converting all the excess to fat? It's all a matter of good carbs versus bad carbs. Your body's self-regulating system works smoothly and efficiently when the carbohydrates you eat come packaged as nature intended—together with the vitamins and minerals required for the metabolism of carbohydrates. The 21-Day Sugar Detox includes only these good carbs, along with quality protein and fat, so you'll be all set while on the program.

The blood sugar balancing act: glucagon at work

You actually have two blood sugar–regulating hormones: insulin and glucagon. Glucagon is the counter-regulatory hormone to insulin—it signals the release of stored glycogen for fuel. Your pancreas releases glucagon in response to three situations: consumption of dense sources of protein (from animal foods), exercise, and hunger. At any given time, one of these two blood sugar–regulating hormones is dominant over the other. In order for your body to be in a releasing or "burning" mode, glucagon needs to be dominant; otherwise, you're in an insulin-dominant storage mode. These two hormones are like the co-directors of the movie that is your metabolism—and there can be only one director in charge at a time on this set.

The response of glucagon to dense protein in the diet is stronger than the release of insulin, so glucagon becomes the dominant hormone over insulin when you eat

increasing glycogen storage capacity

Your glycogen storage space is based primarily on the amount of lean muscle mass you have, but it can be increased if you up the amount of exercise you do, especially at higher intensities. High-intensity exercise gets your heart rate up very high, usually by performing bursts or intervals like sprinting. This does not include steady lower- to moderate-intensity exercise like walking or jogging.

Building more lean muscle mass means that you actually burn more calories all day long, not just when you are huffing and puffing at the gym! You may notice that a lot of athletes not only are able to eat a lot more carbohydrates than those who are less active, but actually *need* to eat those carbohydrates to maintain energy and performance levels. That's because high-intensity exercise demands glucose for fuel. Your body looks for those stored carbohydrates when you hit the peaks of a workout, or even for the duration a very intense workout. So if you try to work out intensely without having stored up some glycogen, you likely won't feel so great. Typical effects of intense exercise without adequate glycogen stores include headache, fatigue, and nausea.

What doesn't demand glucose for fuel? Walking, sitting, standing, light activity, or lower-intensity exercise (like longer-term endurance exercise). In other words, your body functions optimally by burning fat if you are moderately active all day long. ●

a meal higher in protein than carbohydrates. You are able to maintain energy while you exercise thanks to glucagon, which signals the release of glycogen from storage to raise your blood sugar levels to fuel the workout. When you get hungry, glucagon helps out by breaking down stored glycogen into glucose to dump into your bloodstream, keeping you from experiencing a blood sugar crash.

Maintaining even blood sugar levels is the #1 key to fat loss. Even if your primary goal in completing The 21-Day Sugar Detox isn't fat loss, let's be honest: Most of us would be happy to see a little bit of extra body fat disappear. Any time you take in sugar, you raise your blood sugar levels. Doing so puts your body into storage mode versus burning mode—and that often means storing the excess as fat.

CARBS FOR ATHLETES
You may have heard a bit about glycogen stores if you are an athlete, since most athletes need to be acutely aware of how much glycogen they have stored up to use for fueling exercise. Check out the Energy modifications on pages 72, 80, or 88 (depending on your level) to read more about how much carbohydrate athletes should be eating on The 21-Day Sugar Detox. ●

Sugar, stress, and your hormones

Now that you understand a lot more about how sugar and carbohydrates work in your body, let's talk about more reasons why you should avoid bad carbs.

You already know that your food choices impact the blood sugar–regulating hormones insulin and glucagon, but they affect a myriad of other hormones as well. From health challenges like acne, hypothyroidism, polycystic ovarian syndrome (PCOS), low testosterone, or even fertility complications to mood swings, painful periods, or menopause, I always recommend getting blood sugar regulation under control as the first step. What does blood sugar have to do with all of these other hormonal issues? Everything. It's all about stress.

Here's the thing about blood sugar regulation: If it's not working properly, then the rest of your hormonal balance can, and likely will, suffer.

If you eat too many bad carbs and demand lots of insulin to get your blood sugar back to normal, you actually run the risk of feeling that crash of a low blood sugar level. You know that feeling you get 30 minutes to an hour after you indulge in something sweet, or even when you eat too much beans and rice at a Mexican restaurant? You either feel tired, like you could take a nap (a high insulin level), or you feel the crashing effect of the insulin spike that followed your blood sugar spike in an effort to balance you out. In the latter scenario, your blood sugar actually crashes again because the insulin rushed to work so quickly, and you're left feeling shaky, weak, and irritable—and likely looking for more sugar!

Does that sound like a calm situation for your body? You're right, it's not. Both the high level of insulin and the low level of blood sugar are stress-inducing physiological events. In fact, anything that disturbs the inherent desire your body has for internal balance is a stressor.

sugar & inflammation

Inflammation is the body's response to a problem. When your body thinks there's a constant problem, it lives in a chronic state of inflammation. This steady, low level inflammatory state underlies all chronic disease and suppressed immunity. Essentially, it's at the root of just about every disease imaginable. Sugar consumption plays a role in chronic inflammation in two main ways:

1) Depleted nutrient stores from overconsumption of bad carbs lead to a chronic state of stress in the body.

2) Chronically high and/or low blood sugar—what you form when consistently ingesting too many bad carbs or riding the blood sugar roller-coaster—creates a stress state for the body. ●

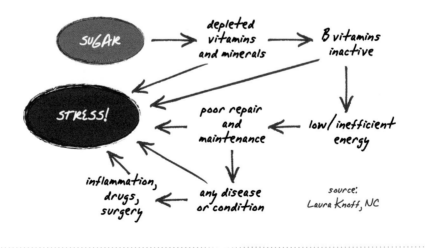

source:
Laura Knoff, NC

The stress hormone cortisol responds to these highs and lows, causing a state of alarm within your body. Cortisol is produced and stored in your adrenal glands, which sit on top of your kidneys. It is often referred to as the fight-or-flight hormone because it's what gets you to take action when you are in danger. You need cortisol just to wake up in the morning and move throughout your day, so having some running through your body is not a bad thing! The problem occurs when it gets out of balance. Too much and you feel on edge; too little and you're dragging, needing caffeine or other stimulants just to function normally.

To better understand the effect cortisol has on your body and its entire hormonal system, it's important to know the way your body releases cortisol in response to stress. When you exercise at a high intensity for a short period, for example, cortisol is released in a controlled, acute fashion—meaning a short, intense burst and then a reprieve. You're quite well equipped to handle this acute phase of stress to your system. Another example would be when you eat a sugary treat on a special occasion, but then return to a whole foods-based diet. Once again, your body experienced an intense burst of stress, and then a reprieve. What you're not well equipped to handle, physiologically, is chronic stress, such as running nonstop for two days straight or drinking a can of soda pop

high or low blood sugar → *cortisol response* → *insulin response to stress*

• WHAT ABOUT DIABETES? •

Without insulin to signal to your cells, they wouldn't receive glucose; it would just stay in your bloodstream, and your blood sugar would skyrocket. An easy way to understand this is to think of people with type 1 diabetes, an autoimmune condition. The beta cells of their pancreas (the cells that make insulin) no longer work to create the hormone. Type 1 diabetics must take shots of insulin so that their cells can receive the glucose that hits their bloodstream; otherwise, their blood sugar could rise to dangerously high, and possibly fatal, levels. The 21DSD lowers carb intake, which is very helpful for type 1 diabetics who are struggling to keep their blood glucose levels down.

In a person with type 2 diabetes, the body still has the ability to make insulin, but the hormone signaling system does not work properly, and the message sent by the insulin to the cells to let glucose in gets garbled. A person with type 2 diabetes may need to take insulin, but the condition is not autoimmune and in most cases can be reversed over time with appropriate diet and lifestyle changes.

Note that The 21DSD is safe for both type 1 and type 2 diabetics, and many have completed the program with great success. If you have either type, you will need to pay special attention to insulin injected, as the dosage may need to be lowered if you reduce your carbohydrate intake while on the program. If you have concerns, consult with your doctor or endocrinologist before you start. ●

every thirty minutes. This produces a daily up-and down of blood sugar and insulin. In regards to food, this is known as the blood sugar roller-coaster.

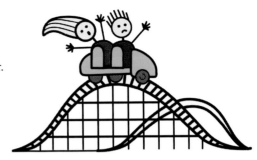

When your body is battling these highs and lows, it's in a constant, low level of that fight-or-flight stress response mode. Let's say that exercise puts your body at a level 8 output of cortisol, and then it recovers to a level 1 of "normal" output so that you can function throughout the day. Riding the blood sugar roller-coaster is like being at level 4 all day long. In the long term, this chronic stress to your system damages your body's ability to respond properly to other stressors.

You already know that excess carbohydrate is stored as fat (triglycerides, body fat, or a combination). What you may not realize is that being in a constant state of stress can also cause your body to store fat, almost regardless of excess carbs or calories. When your body senses chronic stress, which the blood sugar roller-coaster signals, the higher amount of cortisol that your adrenal glands are dishing out actually promotes the storage of body fat. This cortisol-related body fat is typically found around your abdomen and love handle area. So if you're looking to reduce belly fat, getting off the blood sugar roller-coaster and reducing other chronic physical and emotional stressors is critical!

And here's another problem: When the demand for cortisol is abused, your body's ability to produce thyroid and sex hormones is diminished. Your body knows that keeping you alive is more critical than allowing you to maintain a healthy metabolism or to reproduce. So, with this priority, hormones that your body needs to stay balanced with chronic stress are given first dibs, so to speak, at the substrates that are used to make your stress and sex hormones.

Thyroid hormones are known to govern metabolism, and your brain is responsible for sending signals to your thyroid and your adrenal glands at the same time. When a chronic stressor is present, the signaling can run haywire, and your thyroid may suffer. Common symptoms of low thyroid function include fatigue, unexplained weight gain, cold hands and feet, thinning hair, and elevated LDL cholesterol. Many people who've completed The 21DSD program have found that symptoms of an underactive thyroid diminish over the course of the three weeks.

When priority is given to stress hormones for survival, the balance of sex hormone synthesis tends to suffer as well. This is a major reason why so many women experience PMS, painful periods, cramps, and migraines around their cycle.

Hormonal imbalances are all interconnected, and anything that tips you out of balance in one place can cascade into more complex problems elsewhere. Hormonal imbalances can also have direct and significant effects on the appearance and texture of your skin, resulting in acne, psoriasis, and even eczema. Participants on The 21-Day Sugar Detox regularly report significant improvements in all of these skin conditions.

Now that you've learned a lot about what happens in your body when you eat sugar and bad carbs, you can see how important it is to reset your body—and your lifestyle—with The 21-Day Sugar Detox. You'll not only free yourself from cravings, increase energy, and improve sleep and moods, you'll also improve hormonal function and lower inflammation in your body. The positive effects of The 21-Day Sugar Detox are far-reaching—you'll be amazed at the changes you will experience by the end of your three weeks.

This program is straightforward and clear-cut, yes, but the key to making it easy is knowing how to prepare and what to expect. It's not quite as simple as just removing sugar from your diet point-blank. In the following pages, I've outlined steps you can take to gear up for your detox with a simple and effective plan. It will make all the difference to your success!

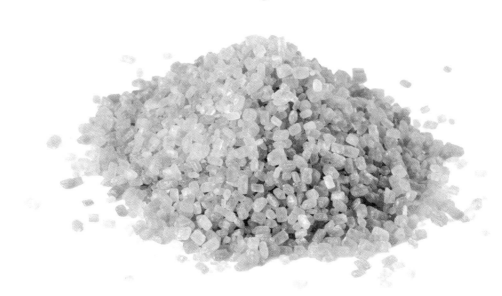

The 21-Day Sugar Detox
preparation checklist

To ensure your success on this program, it's important that you prepare yourself leading up to your start date. Rushing into The 21-Day Sugar Detox is a surefire way to set yourself up for a struggle, whereas preparation and planning will make the experience much smoother and easier for you!

7 DAYS BEFORE DETOX

☐ Understanding what really goes on in your body when you eat sugar and how you benefit when you break the sugar habit will go a long way toward keeping you motivated during the detox and beyond. Read the entire first part of this book through page 61, and review the additional resources in the back of the book beginning on page 220.

☐ Select the level at which you'll be completing the detox, as well as the modifications you'll follow, if necessary (see page 63).

☐ Review the Yes/No lists of foods included in your level of The 21DSD.

☐ Make a list of the foods you currently eat that you'll need to replace while on The 21DSD based on your level/modifications (refer to page 58). If you plan to follow one of the meal plans to the letter, you will not need to complete this step.

☐ If you are following a meal plan from the book, print the corresponding shopping list from the website of both pantry items and fresh items to have on hand.

BALANCEDBITES.COM/21DSD
Printable shopping lists are available online.

☐ Shop for any pantry items you need.

☐ Order pantry items online that you are unable to source locally (see pages 224-225).

☐ Find a friend or family member to join you!

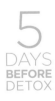

5 DAYS BEFORE DETOX

☐ Check your pantry and fridge for off-plan ingredients and foods. Either plan to finish eating them before you begin, donate them, toss them in the trash, or plan to set them aside somewhere safely out of reach for the duration of your 21DSD.

☐ Seek out alternate grocery store options if you weren't able to stock your pantry at your usual stores—call around to find specific items.

☐ If you think you may want to try some of the supplements listed on pages 40-43, buy them at your local health food store or order them online.

☐ Join and login to the online forum, and/or visit The 21DSD Facebook page to ask questions about replacing foods on your list of swaps if you need help.

FACEBOOK.COM/21DAYSUGARDETOX
Join the conversation.

3 DAYS BEFORE DETOX

- ☐ If you plan to make any of the soup or slow cooker recipes, make the broth on page 212 and freeze portions so that they're ready to go when you need them.

- ☐ Make and bring any dry snacks (nuts, nut butter, jerky, etc.) you've purchased to your workplace so that they're ready to go when you start. (Especially if you start on a Monday. Don't risk forgetting to pack them on Monday morning!) Check out page 184 for a simple jerky recipe.

- ☐ Download and print The 21-Day Sugar Detox Success Log.

  BALANCEDBITES.COM/21DSD
  Download PDFs & sign up for e-mails.

- ☐ Sign up for the free Daily Detox e-mails and select your start date.

1 DAY BEFORE DETOX

- ☐ Triple-check your pantry and fridge to rid them of off-plan items. If you share living or eating space with someone who will not be on The 21DSD with you, create separate shelves in the fridge and pantry so that you know where your food is and are not easily led astray.

- ☐ Have meals planned and/or cooked and ready to go for Day 1! Your biggest key to success is preparation, and Day 1 success will catapult you forward.

- ☐ Begin filling in The 21-Day Sugar Detox Daily Success Log with Day 0—the day before you start your 21DSD!

what to expect, day-by-day

a look at what your 21 days may feel like,
and what to do about it

It's always good to go into something new knowing what you can expect, so I'm going to walk you through some of the feelings you might have while on The 21DSD—both physical and mental. Your experience may vary by a day or two here or there. You may not encounter many of the tougher times that I'm going to describe, or your experience may come with a few more bumps in the road. This timeline is based on feedback from thousands of participants who've completed the program over the last several years, but realize that your exact day-by-day detox will be unique to you! For example, if you are not exercising while on The 21DSD, the days that cover how you may feel during a workout will clearly not apply. You'll notice that some days seem overwhelmingly positive, upbeat, and like you are on top of the world, while other days seem to be much more of a struggle. This fluctuation of feelings is normal and expected! Rest assured that as you finish out the three weeks, your physical and emotional state will be strong. On Day 21, you'll feel like a champ!

DAY 0 "HERE WE GO!"

You may experience: Anxiety, excitement, fear, or busyness as you prepare.

Your best bet is to: Approach your 21DSD feeling hopeful and positive. A good attitude is the best foundation, along with all the planning and prep you have done. If you haven't gone through the Preparation Checklist on page 32, get to it! It gives preparation tips for the seven days before you start the program.

DAY 1 "I GOT THIS!"

You may experience: No effects at all, or possibly some extremely strong cravings. You may feel extra hungry (this is why I remind you that this isn't a diet and that if you are hungry, you should eat from your Yes foods list!), or you may feel like you are eating a lot. This new approach may mean eating a lot more food than you're used to—and that's okay!

Your best bet is to: Roll with the positivity that Day 1 brings.

DAY 2 "THIS ISN'T SO BAD." OR "WILL THIS GET EASIER?!"

You may experience: No symptoms at all, or headaches, mental fogginess, or hunger.

Your best bet is to: Keep trucking! Make sure that your meals are well balanced with enough protein and fat, along with the appropriate carbs according to your level or modifications.

DAY 3 "AM I GOING TO MAKE IT THROUGH THIS?"

You may experience: Fatigue, cold- and flu-like symptoms, low blood sugar, or self-doubt. Day 3 is the beginning of some of the hardest days for most folks!

Your best bet is to: Realize that you are not likely experiencing a "real" cold or flu, but the effects of detoxing from sugar. Be careful not to rush off to the doctor; just know that this reaction is common and will subside within a few days. Focus on the positives that are ahead—liberation from your cravings and a healthier you inside and out.

DAY 4 "THREE DAYS DOWN, EIGHTEEN TO GO!"

You may experience: Mood changes, minor skin irritation, or breakouts. Acne is a common detox symptom and is a great sign that your body is working to clear toxins!

Your best bet is to: Remember that awareness is key when it comes to your mood. Try not to react to those around you in a hypersensitive way and remember that the change in your diet is likely affecting your mood more than you realize. For your skin, add milk thistle (tea, tincture, or capsules) and ginger tea to aid in detoxification. Take care to read the ingredients in products you apply to your skin, as they may cause further irritation. I highly recommend the oil cleansing method (OCM).

DAY 5 "OKAY, I'M GETTING THE HANG OF THIS."

You may experience: Headaches starting to clear and fewer cravings, or struggles with temptation and slip-ups if you're unprepared and hunger sets in.

Your best bet is to: Remember what got you off on the right foot in the first place: preparation! That early start you had to getting food ready, having healthy snacks on hand, and planning meals was right on, and now you may need to revisit that preparation. Take action, and make sure that you have 21DSD-friendly meals and snacks ready to go.

OCM 4-1-1
Want to know more about oil cleansing and other natural skincare salvation? I highly recommend the *Skintervention Guide* by Liz Wolfe. You can find out more about the guide and other skincare tips at balancedbites.com/21DSD.

DAY 6 "HOW CAN I MAKE WEEK 2 AS SUCCESSFUL AS WEEK 1?"

You may experience: Cold- or flu-like symptoms beginning to subside.

Your best bet is to: Revisit your meal planning outline, and be sure that you are ready for Week 2 before it starts.

DAY 7 "WOW, ALMOST A WHOLE WEEK DOWN. I FEEL AWESOME! BUT MY DIGESTION, NOT SO MUCH."

You may experience: Digestive issues such as bloating, constipation, or diarrhea. These symptoms may be discouraging, but there's hope!

Your best bet is to: Check out the FAQ section (see page 51). We've got your digestion covered!

DAY 8 "TWO MORE WEEKS...I WANT A COOKIE!"

You may experience: A slip-up or temptation to eat off-plan foods over the weekend; guilt over having had a slip-up. Fatigue can also kick in at this point if you didn't experience it very early on.

Your best bet is to: Don't beat yourself up over a slip-up, whether you realized it was happening or not. A slip-up doesn't define you or your entire experience, though it should be a wake-up call that you need to recommit yourself to your plan and to yourself. You deserve to get through this simple three-week program on track! But, hey, you can always have a 21DSD-friendly cookie. Check out the recipe on page 195.

DAY 9 "I'M GETTING TIRED OF THE FOOD I'M EATING!"

You may experience: Being overwhelmed by how much time is involved in food prep.

Your best bet is to: Remember that there are tons of easy recipes right here in this book and in your meal plan, along with countless 21DSD-friendly recipes accessible online. Your free Daily Detox e-mails will link to lots of them, so don't forget to click through for ideas. Visit balancedbites.com/21DSD for even more resources and links!

DAY 10 "ALMOST HALFWAY THERE AND I'M FEELING GOOD!"

You may experience: Digestive issues such as gas and bloating (if you had them) clearing up. You're getting the swing of cooking, and you have collected a bunch of recipes to try.

Your best bet is to: Make some new shopping lists and try a new recipe! If you neglected Week 2 shopping and prep, get back into it now. If you have clipped some recipes from outside of this book, add them to your meal plans and buy the ingredients.

DAY 11 "I CAN'T BELIEVE I'M NOT CRAVING SUGAR RIGHT NOW!"

You may experience: An acute awareness of how food was making you feel before The 21DSD; surprise that you aren't noticing many cravings anymore.

Your best bet is to: Make some notes about how you're feeling and recount to yourself some of the struggles and successes you've experienced. Take advantage of the daily success log available at balancedbites.com/21DSD (sample on pages 56-57)—download it and start filling it in now if you haven't already!

DAY 12 "I'M NOT FEELING AS STRONG IN MY WORKOUTS."

You may experience: Shakiness or weakness from going too low-carb; athletes may not be performing as well (especially if not doing modifications). If you're working out regularly (and if you are, you know you should be following the Energy modifications, right?), it's around this time that you may notice your workouts suffering if you haven't remembered to add those dense carb sources to your meals.

Your best bet is to: Revisit the meal plan recommendations and make sure that you're adding the appropriate carb sources to your post-workout meals per the Energy modifications notes that correspond to your level (also see pages 220-221).

DAY 13 "THIS REALLY ISN'T SO HARD. MAYBE I SHOULD EAT THIS WAY ALL THE TIME."

You may experience: Noticeable improvements in mood and energy as you approach the end of your second week.

Your best bet is to: Ride the wave! Share your experience with others and think about how you feel, the healthy choices you're making, and how much you've learned.

DAY 14 "I'M SLEEPING LIKE A BABY—IS THIS FOR REAL?"

You may experience: Not only falling asleep faster, but also sleeping better through the night and waking up feeling more well rested.

Your best bet is to: Continue to cultivate good sleep habits (getting to bed and waking up at consistent times daily; sleeping in a dark, cool room; and creating a nightly ritual) to ensure that you get enough sleep through the rest of the detox and beyond.

DAY 15 "NOT. ANOTHER. GREEN. APPLE."

You may experience: Boredom with food choices and longings for foods that you have eliminated. At first you were pretty excited about the fact that you could make it through 21 days with at least some fruit. By now, however, your giddiness over a green apple or an underripe banana may have faded.

Your best bet is to: Stop just *looking* at all the recipes in this book, the recipes sent to your Daily Detox e-mails, and the recipes spread all over Pinterest; go get the ingredients and make them! Some people think that narrowing food choices limits what you can eat, but the number of 21DSD-friendly recipes out there is virtually limitless if you just look around. Check out the resources on page 223 for more 21DSD-friendly recipes than you can eat in three weeks. Or even in a year!

DAY 16 "I KNOW THIS ISN'T A WEIGHT-LOSS PLAN, BUT I WAS SECRETLY HOPING THAT I WOULD LOSE SOME WEIGHT!"

You may experience: Some movement on the scale or extra room in your clothes (even better). But you may not. It's best not to get on the scale except once before and once after your 21DSD—otherwise, you'll drive yourself crazy watching those numbers.

Your best bet is to: Step away from the scale. Review the many reasons why you decided to begin this detox in the first place, and focus on the amazing changes that have happened in your body and your life so far.

DAY 17 "ARE WE THERE YET?!?"

You may experience: Feelings of impatience for the end of the detox. Day 17 is almost like "hump day" on The 21DSD.

Your best bet is to: Keep checking in with friends who are on the detox with you and with supporters you've met online. Think of a non-food reward that you'll "win" at the end of the 21 days—buy that cookbook you've had your eye on, get a manicure, treat yourself to a day at a museum, go to a play or concert, buy tickets to a sporting event, or outfit your kitchen with some new tools.

DAY 18 "I REALLY AM IN THE HOME STRETCH NOW, BUT WHAT AM I GOING TO DO AFTER THIS?"

You may experience: Some anxiety about what you'll do after the 21 days are up—this is normal.

Your best bet is to: Check out the advice in "After The 21-Day Sugar Detox" on pages 53-55.

DAY 19 "THIS IS CLOSE ENOUGH TO 21 DAYS, RIGHT? A LITTLE BITE OF [INSERT FOOD YOU'VE BEEN MISSING HERE] WON'T HURT, WILL IT?"

You may experience: A strong urge to "cheat" or call it good enough at 19 days.

Your best bet is to: Keep your eyes on the prize. Remember that this detox is not just about getting sugar out of your life for three weeks; it's also about changing your habits. When you make it through just three more days, the feeling of accomplishment will be awesome!

DAY 20 "ON DAY 22, I'M GOING TO GO CRAZY AND EAT EVERYTHING I WANT!"

You may experience: A strong desire to plan an all-out carb-fest.

Your best bet is to: Focus on these last two days, and finish up strong! Worry about Day 22 when it comes, not today!

DAY 21 "THIS IS IT!"

You may experience: Relief, pride, excitement, and sheer joy that you made it to Day 21!

Your best bet is to: Finish this day out strong. Get your head on straight about what tomorrow will bring, and review page 53-55 for advice on what to do after you complete the program!

DAY 22 "I DID IT! PASS THE CHOCOLATE!"

You may experience: Apprehension about adding foods that were on the No list for the last three weeks back to your regular diet.

Your best bet is to: Take it easy! Go slowly, and add back foods little by little. A bender on a bunch of sugary foods will almost always leave you feeling very sick!

supplement recommendations

"The individual who says it is not possible should move out of the way of those doing it." —Tricia Cunningham

Once you start The 21-Day Sugar Detox, you may wonder if there is anything that can help with the cravings you may be experiencing. I always recommend that you try natural, food-based approaches to curbing cravings before you look to herbal or vitamin and mineral supplements for support. Two great solutions are:

• Lemon water (sometimes with L-glutamine added; see below). Hydrating with a hint of flavor from lemon or other citrus can help with that urge to grab something sweet.

• Herbal teas (sometimes with a touch of full-fat coconut milk added). I love the Traditional Medicinals brand of organic teas. Here are some varieties that you may want to try: Ginger, Peppermint, Think O2, Licorice root (drink it only before 3pm, as it can have a stimulating effect).

Herbal teas support different body systems, so read the descriptions to find out more. That said, tea's "medicinal" properties are typically pretty mild, so you needn't be concerned that a tea has specific properties if you love to drink it simply for its flavor. Keep in mind that it is often better to use one tea bag for multiple cups of tea so that the strength is diluted over time, instead of drinking very potent tea all day.

If water and tea don't lessen your cravings, you can try a few different herbs and supplements to help yourself out. Everybody is unique and will respond differently to them, but they're all pretty mild and should have only beneficial effects in the moderate dosages recommended here.

With all of the dosage recommendations, more does not necessarily mean better. It is always best to start out at a low dose so that you can see how your system responds for a few days. I've listed my recommendations here in the order that I recommend trying them, with cinnamon as the #1 supplemental super-spice I'd add to your food while on The 21DSD.

DISCLAIMER

If you are taking medications, are pregnant or nursing, or have a diagnosed or serious medical condition, please consult with your physician, naturopath, or other healthcare professional before beginning any new supplements. ●

CINNAMON

WHAT IS IT? An aromatic spice.

WHAT DOES IT DO? Cinnamon helps regulate blood sugar while creating a bit of a sensation that you're eating something sweet, giving the satisfaction of a treat without triggering your body's sweet-taste response. According to whfoods.com, "Cinnamon slows the rate at which the stomach empties after meals, reducing the rise in blood sugar after eating."

HOW MUCH SHOULD I TAKE? You can add as much cinnamon as you like to the foods you eat, or sprinkle it in tea or coffee. Add up to 1 1/2 teaspoons to full-fat coconut or almond milk–based smoothies following the recipes in this book. You may also decide to make one of the sweetener-free treat recipes and add cinnamon according to your taste preferences. Cinnamon can also be paired with other flavorings, like curry or chili powder, to season meats—especially pork chops, ground beef, or lamb—and create a sweet and savory dish.

WHEN SHOULD I TAKE IT? Feel free to enjoy cinnamon on foods at any time of day. Many of the treat recipes in this book include cinnamon.

L-GLUTAMINE

WHAT IS IT? An amino acid. Dietary sources of L-glutamine include high-protein foods like beef, chicken, fish, and eggs. This supplement tends to be far more effective at battling cravings when taken in conjunction with a diet rich in these foods.

WHAT DOES IT DO? L-glutamine supports the repair of the gut lining (small intestines) and improves gut function, which will always help regulate your body's systems, including metabolism and cravings. It also helps reduce sugar cravings by providing energy to cells.

HOW MUCH SHOULD I TAKE? 2 to 4 grams in water up to twice a day in powder form. If you experience any constipation after adding L-glutamine to your daily routine, stop taking it until your eliminations become regular again, then resume it at half the dose.

WHEN SHOULD I TAKE IT? Between meals, beginning as early and ending as late in the day as you like.

MAGNESIUM

WHAT IS IT? A mineral. Dietary sources include kelp, pumpkin seeds, sunflower seeds, spinach, broccoli, Swiss chard, salmon, oysters, halibut, scallops, dried herbs, and bone broth.

WHAT DOES IT DO? Magnesium plays a role in more than 300 enzymatic processes in the body, and it has a particularly important role in powering energy production (cellular energy, as you learned about earlier). It also helps insulin take action appropriately; blood sugar management is much easier when you get enough magnesium.

HOW MUCH SHOULD I TAKE? Option 1: 300 to 600 milligrams a day of Natural Calm powdered drink mix (magnesium citrate). You can use 1/2 teaspoon to begin and go up from there if needed. People who weigh less than 130 pounds should take the lower end of the range. If you experience loose stools after taking a dose, you took too much and should take less the next time. Note: This product is very sweet, but if you overdo it, you'll feel some negative effects, so I am not overly concerned with the sweetness being an issue. Take this supplement no more than once per day. Option 2: 300 to 600 milligrams a day of magnesium glycinate or magnesium malate in capsule form.

WHEN SHOULD I TAKE IT? Magnesium can be taken at any time of day, but it can have a relaxing effect, so you may find that taking it in the evening after dinner is ideal.

CHROMIUM

WHAT IS IT? A mineral that can be found on shelves as chromium picolinate, polynicotinate, and Chelavite. Dietary sources include eggs, onions, romaine lettuce, ripe tomatoes, liver, peppers, green apples with peel, and sea vegetables like nori (dried seaweed paper), kelp, and dulse.

WHAT DOES IT DO? Chromium helps increase insulin sensitivity, which affects how well your body regulates its blood sugar levels. According to naturopath Michael Murray, "Chromium supplementation is indicated in both diabetes and hypoglycemia because of its ability to improve blood sugar control."

HOW MUCH SHOULD I TAKE? 200 micrograms one to three times a day (a total of 200 to 600 micrograms).

WHEN SHOULD I TAKE IT? 200 micrograms at a time with meals. If you are taking one or two doses a day, take them with breakfast and lunch and not with dinner.

B VITAMINS

WHAT IS IT? Water-soluble vitamins. Dietary sources of B vitamins include liver, dairy (if you are eating raw/unpasteurized or organic full-fat dairy), leafy greens, eggs, and meats (which mainly provide B12).

WHAT DOES IT DO? B vitamins play an important role in the complex process of cell metabolism. They help combat fatigue and are often lacking from the diet.

HOW MUCH SHOULD I TAKE? 100 milligrams twice a day of vitamin B complex.

WHEN SHOULD I TAKE IT? Take vitamin B complex with breakfast and lunch. B vitamins often give the sensation of an energy boost, so it's best to avoid them in the evening.

GYMNEMA

WHAT IS IT? An herb also known as gymnema sylvestre. You may find it in capsule, tablet, powder, or liquid form. If you can find the leaves, you may chew on them or steep them with your herbal tea.

WHAT DOES IT DO? Gymnema can reduce the taste of sugar when it's placed in the mouth, thereby assisting in limiting your sugar cravings.

HOW MUCH SHOULD I TAKE? Follow the dosage instructions on the package you buy, and start out slowly. Try one dose and go from there based on how you feel.

WHEN SHOULD I TAKE IT? Any time you anticipate a craving, or whenever you drink an herbal tea from which you don't want to experience sweetness.

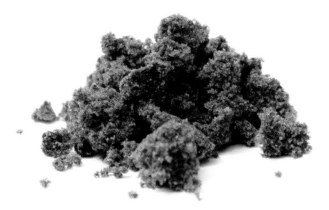

frequently asked questions

"By failing to prepare, you are preparing to fail."

—Benjamin Franklin

THE PROGRAM

How is The 21-Day Sugar Detox different from other nutrition challenges, detoxes, and cleanse programs out there?

Many nutrition challenges take a general approach to helping you eat better, get healthier, or lose weight. That's great! The 21-Day Sugar Detox actually does all that, but its main goal is to help you bust sugar and carb cravings. This program is specifically focused on directing your tastes and habits away from sweet foods. The amazing thing is, many of the natural foods you'll enjoy on the program will taste very sweet after a few days away from sugar and refined foods! There are no required shakes, powders, potions, or pills, though there are some smoothie recipes that you are welcome to enjoy if you choose (see page 92), and some supplements that may be helpful (see page 40). This is not a vegetarian program or a program that relies on complicated recipes or deprivation for success. If you are hungry on The 21DSD, you can eat from a huge list of plant and animal foods. You may experience a few rocky days while your body transitions off of sugar, but for the most part, it will get easier as the days pass.

Can't I just eliminate all sugar from my diet and complete a "sugar detox" on my own without this program?

Yes and no. It may seem obvious that simply removing sugar is an "easy" way to detox. But the not-so-simple part is that just removing sugar doesn't always get rid of the cravings. Having a more complete picture of which foods contain sugar, act like sugar in the body, and trigger cravings is a critical element of success on this program. I created The 21DSD to help people who find the prospect of removing sugar from their diets daunting and want to follow a guided, supportive, and clear-cut plan that encompasses more. Many people find that it's tough to figure out the best approach to curbing cravings, and that removing sugar in obvious forms doesn't go far enough. It's great to be able to answer this question, by the way, because it's one that you are likely to be asked while you're on The 21DSD!

Is this a low-carb, zero-carb, or zero-sugar program?

Not even close! The 21-Day Sugar Detox eliminates all added sugars, sweeteners, and refined foods, but it includes plenty of real-food carbohydrate sources as well as some natural sugars from whole foods. The amount of carbs and foods containing natural sugars (like full-fat dairy and limited fruit) you will eat on the program will be based on your specific needs and activity levels. For example, you may find that you need the Energy modifications, which add more whole-food, dense-carb sources to help fuel your body for things like exercising or nursing a young one.

Can I complete The 21-Day Sugar Detox more than once?

Absolutely! Many people come back to the program more than once a year, often to complete it at a higher level or with a different focus than the previous time. Some people take just a week or so off at the end of the first 21 days, and then begin again with the groups that start on the first Monday of each month. Other people find that simply rolling their 21 days into 30 or more days works for them.

I've heard that detoxing isn't recommended for pregnant or breastfeeding moms. Is The 21DSD safe for these moms?

Yes! While it may be true that some detox protocols are not recommended for women who are pregnant or breastfeeding, The 21DSD is simply a whole foods–based program. It is not designed to clear specific toxins, such as heavy metals or other impurities, from your system by using supplements. That isn't what The 21DSD is about. In fact, many pregnant and breastfeeding moms have already completed the program with great success, often finding that they can avoid the problems with gestational diabetes that they experienced in previous pregnancies. This program has you eating real, whole, natural foods—it's that simple. That approach is healthy for everyone, pregnant, breastfeeding, or otherwise. If you are pregnant or breastfeeding, you should follow the Energy modifications for whichever level of the program you choose to complete. The Energy modifications will direct you to eat more carb-dense foods than are typically included for others on the level you've selected. For example, you'll add more sweet potatoes to meals. This will help you feel more energized as well as support a healthy milk supply.

Is it safe to eat this way all the time?

The 21DSD is a low-sugar, low-trigger-foods diet. It is not only a perfectly safe way to eat; it's a fantastic way to eat in the long term. It isn't really a diet at all; it's a lifestyle. Eating real, whole foods is always safe and healthy. A large majority of people keep their bad-carb-free ways intact after the program because they learn how much better they feel without them. Here are some ways that people transition their sugar detox into a way of eating that feels a bit easier and more manageable for them:

- add a serving or two of seasonal fruits each day

- add a square or two of organic 85% dark chocolate

- add more good carbs in the form of starchier foods like sweet potato or plantains (if these weren't included in recommended modifications to the program)

- research ways of eating that are quite similar to The 21DSD, such as Paleo, primal, or grain-free approaches

Is there anyone who shouldn't complete The 21DSD?

I don't recommend that you begin the program if you are currently training for an all-day athletic competition (for example, a CrossFit competition), a marathon, or any other type of endurance event that will take more than an hour to complete. I suggest that you wait until both your training and the event are complete. You can fuel your body for everyday training and shorter-duration competitive events or races by following the Energy modifications while on The 21DSD.

Is The 21DSD appropriate as an anti-Candida diet?

The 21DSD is not specifically designed as a Candida overgrowth (Candidiasis) detox program and should not be considered a substitute for a professional medical diagnosis or treatment. If you have been diagnosed with Candidiasis, you may notice that the foods you eat and avoid on The 21DSD are very well aligned with many programs that are created specifically to target the die-off of the *Candida albicans* fungus.

The following are symptoms of Candida die-off, but you may also feel them as a result of the change in fuel you are putting into your body while on The 21DSD (that is, more fat instead of more carbs): nausea, headache, fatigue, dizziness, swollen glands, cold-like symptoms, bloating, gas, constipation or diarrhea, skin rashes or breakouts, sweating, fever, and recurring vaginal or sinus infections. These symptoms are also known as *carb-flu* and should not be used to reach a diagnosis of Candidiasis.

Unlike The 21DSD, most specifically anti-Candida diet protocols eliminate all fermented foods. If you suspect that you may have Candidiasis (if the above-listed symptoms persist for more than a week), you may want to avoid sauerkraut, kombucha, aged cheeses, and yogurt or kefir, along with all other fermented foods, for your 21DSD.

If you suspect you are suffering from Candidiasis, I highly recommend working with a naturopath or other healthcare practitioner to diagnose and treat the infection. Additionally, experiencing symptoms of Candida die-off for more than two weeks while on The 21DSD is uncommon and may indicate a different underlying health concern. If this sounds like your experience, I recommend that you find a healthcare practitioner to work with you on your health challenges.

Can I modify the program to suit my own needs?

I would never tell you that customizing a plan to suit your needs is a bad idea—that's entirely up to you. I will say, however, that if you haven't completed the program as written for at least three weeks (at whichever level you choose), then I strongly urge you to do so before making any changes. Many people who tailor the program outside of the written guidelines don't find the same success as those who follow it as written. That said, since this program is entirely about eating real, whole foods, if you find another route that works better for you after you have completed this program as written at least once, I invite you to use that route instead!

THE FOOD

Why are some fruits included in the program while others aren't? Don't some fruits that are off-plan actually have less sugar than the included fruits?

The primary goal of The 21DSD is to change your palate and your habits, so I'm taking you out of your comfort zone by allowing only fairly bitter, sour, and bland fruits, such as green apples, underripe bananas, and grapefruit. While the natural sugar content of some of the included fruits is in fact higher than that of, say, berries, the included fruits don't tend to taste very sweet or trigger further cravings for sugar.

I'm worried that eating fruits will trigger my sugar cravings. Can I limit fruits even further than the program recommends?

I don't recommend that you attempt to limit fruits further than the program already outlines. Thousands of participants who've included these limited fruits feel that they provide a small relief from the stress of being overly restricted, but they don't result in the urge to overindulge as very sweet fruits like mango and pineapple can. This is one of those "don't be a hero" points that I want you to understand: Eliminating the allowed fruits doesn't make the program more effective simply because it reduces sugars further. The only reason eliminating these fruits would be beneficial to your success is if you found that your habits around them were becoming unhealthy. Including one piece of the allowed fruit, in whatever form you choose—baked, sautéed, raw, with a nut butter, or over a salad—is entirely up to you. I invite you to enjoy these whole, natural foods if they feel good for you. However, if you find that your habits around their consumption become unhealthy, you can make the call to limit them for yourself.

Why are some nuts included in the program while others aren't?

Cashews and peanuts are out for The 21DSD, while other nuts are Yes foods. As I mentioned in the response to the limited fruits question above, one goal of the program is to change your palate and habits. Cashews tend to trigger sweet-taste habits and become hard to limit, so they are out. Peanuts are known to carry high levels of aflatoxin, a type of mold that can develop in foods like grains and legumes. Because this is a detox program, it excludes peanuts for this known toxin-load issue.

I'm on Level 3. What can I put in my coffee since dairy is on my No list?

If you absolutely can't drink your coffee black, I recommend the following options:

1. Organic, full-fat (not light) coconut milk from a can (my top pick). Good brands include Whole Foods, Thai Kitchen, Native Forest (BPA-free cans), and Natural Value (BPA-free cans, no guar gum additive).

2. Almond milk. Watch out for additives like carrageenan, "natural flavors," citric acid, and sweeteners. Get unsweetened varieties without additives, or make your own quite easily from whole raw almonds (see the recipe on page 213).

3. Butter from grass-fed cows. Simply whip the butter (the only dairy allowed on Level 3) into warm or hot coffee with a blender, and it becomes creamy and frothy. Grass-fed brands include KerryGold, SMJÖR, Organic Valley Pasture Butter, Kalona Supernatural, and Natural by Nature.

What can I drink besides water?

I love to squeeze lemon or lime into fresh water, or even add some cucumber slices for a "spa water" feel. You can also drink bubbly mineral water (brands like San Pellegrino or Gerolsteiner are great) and seltzer water, but not brands that include "natural flavors" or sweeteners. Herbal teas are a great option for all day; just watch out for sneaky ingredients. Look for organic varieties, as they tend to have fewer additives; Traditional Medicinals is a great brand. You can also enjoy green tea, white tea, black tea, and coffee, but these are not recommended after noon since the caffeine may interfere with sleep.

What sauces and dressings can I use?

There are several recipes in this book that are perfect for all levels, and many more are linked to on the resources page at balancedbites.com/21DSD. Most store-bought and restaurant sauces and dressings have added sugars or sweeteners. Crazy, right? But it's true. Turn a bottle around the next time you pick one up, and read the ingredients.

Can I eat bacon and other cured meats on The 21DSD?

Yes! Sugar will nearly always be listed in the ingredients, but this is an exception to the no-sugar/no-sweeteners rule. When sugar is used in the cure, it isn't actually left in the resulting bacon. What you want to avoid when buying bacon are preservatives like BHA, BHT, sodium phosphates, sodium ascorbate, and anything else you can't pronounce! It's not critical to eat nitrate-free bacon, but the types of nitrate that are natural and okay to eat are celery salt and beet juice.

What are FODMAPs? Who should avoid them?

FODMAP is an acronym that stands for "fermentable oligosaccharides, disaccharides, monosaccharides, and polyols." These are types of carbohydrates that can be difficult for some people to digest, resulting in symptoms varying from gas and bloating to diarrhea, constipation, or a combination or alternation of the two. Unlike foods that can't be tolerated as a result of incomplete digestion within the small intestine, FODMAP foods become irritating to people for the following reasons:

- Overgrowth of the wrong type of bacteria in the system (dysbiosis)

- Overgrowth of bacteria in the wrong part of the digestive system, usually the small intestine, where bacteria don't normally live (this condition is known as small intestinal bacterial overgrowth, or SIBO)

- Low stomach acid production or secretion, which also contributes to the previous two bacterial issues

- A gut pathogen or infection often acquired during travel abroad

If a recipe calls for ingredients containing FODMAPs, it will be highlighted in the list of potentially problematic ingredients. If the recipe can be made without those ingredients, an ingredient tip will suggest omitting them. For example, a recipe may read "FODMAP FREE? Omit the shallots." If you find that you react to these foods, I recommend working with a naturopath, chiropractor, or other practitioner who can submit stool tests to a lab for analysis in order to determine the root cause of the intolerance.

To learn more about digestion, how it should work, and what to do when things go wrong, check out my book *Practical Paleo*.

What are nightshades? Who should avoid them?

Nightshades are a family of plants that contain specific alkaloid compounds that can be irritating to those suffering from joint pain and inflammation. Tomatoes, white potatoes, peppers (bell and hot), and eggplant are the most commonly consumed nightshades. Black pepper and sweet potatoes are not nightshades, however. Note that if a packaged food names "spices" as an ingredient without listing which specific ones are included, paprika is probably one of them. People who are sensitive to nightshades should avoid these items since paprika is derived from peppers. Some other, less frequently consumed nightshades include tomatillos, goji berries, cape gooseberries (but not normal gooseberries), ground cherries (but not Bing or Rainier cherries), garden huckleberries (but not blueberries), and ashwagandha (an herb), as well as tobacco. If you suffer from joint pain or inflammation, arthritis, cracking, or any other joint-related issues, you may choose to eliminate nightshades from your diet for the duration of The 21DSD as well.

If a recipe calls for nightshade foods, it will be highlighted in the list of potentially problematic ingredients. If the recipe can be made without those ingredients, an ingredient tip will suggest omitting them. For example, a recipe may read "NIGHTSHADE FREE? Omit the paprika." If you find that you react to these foods, I recommend working with a naturopath, chiropractor, or other practitioner who can submit stool tests to a lab for analysis in order to determine the root cause of the intolerance.

YOUR BODY

Will I lose weight on The 21DSD?

I recommend that you do not weigh yourself while on the program. You may weigh yourself before you start, and then again after your 21 days are up, but not in between. Your energy, your mood, and even how your clothes fit are far better indicators of health. While a large portion of participants do report weight loss on The 21DSD, it isn't the main focus of the program, and you may not experience the same results as others.

I've noticed some changes to my digestion; is this normal? What can I do to alleviate these problems?

If you experience constipation while on The 21DSD, I highly recommend adding some fermented foods like raw sauerkraut (sold in the refrigerated section at grocery stores; see page 224 for brands), kombucha (up to 8 ounces per day), or fermented pickles. It's also important to get a bit more soluble fiber into your diet if you are constipated. Soluble fiber can come from foods like carrots, parsnips, or butternut squash. If you are following the Energy modifications, sweet potato is a good choice for soluble fiber.

If you find that your eliminations are looser or more frequent than usual while on The 21DSD, adding a cup or more per day of Bone Broth (recipe on page 212) and/or supplementing with L-glutamine as outlined on page 41 can be quite helpful. Avoid leafy greens, like kale and collards, as well as nuts and seeds if your digestion seems to be irritated and moving more quickly than normal.

For a more complete description of support for digestive concerns, please visit The 21DSD resources page at balancedbites.com/21DSD.

THE SUPPLEMENTS

Do I have to take the supplements recommended on pages 40-43 to be successful on The 21DSD?

Absolutely not! I provide a list of supplements to serve as additional support based on both what I know will be helpful and the feedback that thousands of people have provided over the years. Feel free to start using them at any time in your program, or ignore them completely.

If I decide to try some of the supplements, where can I find brands that you recommend?

Visit balancedbites.com/21DSD to find links to the products I recommend.

• I WANT CANDY... •

I don't recommend candy as part of your healthy lifestyle choices post-21DSD. Instead, choose fresh or dried fruits like mango or pineapple, which are quite sweet and far superior to candy when you have your Sugar Monster under control but feel like a sweet treat is in order. ●

MINDSET & HABITS

Am I weak for needing this detox? Why isn't relying on willpower enough to kick my cravings?

Many people seem to rely on self-control, assuming that we are stronger than the foods that surround us, and that we can make deliberate choices and always pick what's healthiest. The problem is our instincts tend to push us in a different direction. Do you think that our prehistoric ancestors would have walked past some berries growing on a bush or some ripe fruit growing in a tree, or would have passed

Are moderation and self-control myths?

You may notice that this book contains recipes for treats. "Doesn't the idea of giving myself a treat run counter to this whole idea of changing my habits?" you might be wondering. Well, I've found that for some people, being allowed small indulgences makes it easier to stick with the program. Whether or not you will be able to eat only small to moderate amounts of something you know can be problematic for you in larger amounts is not something I can answer for you. It may be that even a small taste of something sweet will turn you into a Sugar Monster, searching every corner in your house for anything and everything sweet and stopping at nothing until you have eaten all that you find. Or it may be that a small taste of a healthy sweet treat will quell your craving, and you will be able to move on with your day. Understanding your own habits and behavior patterns is critical to your success in eliminating excess sugar from your diet during The 21DSD and, more importantly, after your three-week detox.

Here's a short quiz to help you evaluate your capacity for moderation and self-control:

1. Are you unable to have just one bite or one portion of a food that you feel you shouldn't eat?

2. Do you find yourself consistently looking to replace treats from your previous eating habits with healthier alternatives?

3. If there are treats near you in your home or office, do you find it impossible to resist them?

4. Do you consider yourself someone with zero willpower?

If you answered Yes to any of these questions, then perhaps making 21DSD-friendly treats won't be a good approach for you. To find out whether it's the sugar in the treats causing you to lose control or it's just the idea that you want a treat, bring a little self-testing into play. I recommend that you make something from the recipes in this book that seems like a treat and see how you do with it. If you're able to eat a portion and leave the rest for another day or for someone else to enjoy, great! If you find that you're unable to control yourself around these foods, then you may want to address why you have an emotional attachment to soothing foods.

up the chance to score some honey from a nearby hive? No way. Now, how sweet natural foods were long ago is not even close to what we experience in our modern, processed food–filled world, but the instinct remains. If there are sweets nearby, we want to eat them. We are entirely capable of training our minds and our habits to keep us from falling prey to these instincts, but we have to work at it. That's what The 21-Day Sugar Detox is all about!

THE SUPPORT

I don't think I can do this on my own! Where can I find support from others who are trying to kick their sugar habits?

One of my favorite things about this program is that the community is huge—and growing every day! We have tens of thousands of current and past program participants on The 21DSD Facebook page (facebook.com/21daysugardetox) as well as on the forums talking about The 21DSD (balancedbites.com/forums). You are never alone while on this program. Every day new people are starting out. A new group starts on the first Monday of each month if you'd like to join a group that will be on the same day of the detox with you. You can also sign up for the free Daily Detox e-mails on the website, which include video links of previous participants sharing their stories and helping others along the way.

I'd like to read more about sugar's effects on my body. What other reading/resources would you recommend?

My first book, *Practical Paleo*
Protein Power Life Plan by Drs. Michael R. Eades and Mary Dan Eades
Sweet Deception by Dr. Joseph Mercola
Naked Calories by Dr. Jayson Calton and Mira Calton
Sugar Blues by William Duffy
Sugar Nation by Jeff O'Connell
The Blood Sugar Solution by Dr. Mark Hyman

What should I do after The 21-Day Sugar Detox?

It's Day 22, and you're thinking with excitement about all the things you haven't eaten for three weeks and that you want to eat all at once.

Stop right there! I highly advise that you pause and reflect on the following points before chugging a glass of fruit juice or scarfing down a pile of candy, some cookies, or even a piece of pizza:

- Do you see now how your diet before The 21-Day Sugar Detox was filled with bad carbs, added sugars, or trigger foods that make you spiral into eating more and more?

- How do you feel now that you've reduced the amount of sugar or bad carbs you eat?

- How has your sleep been? What about your digestive function?

- Do you think that eating sugary or carb-rich foods will make you feel better or worse?

- Has the time and energy commitment that you've put into avoiding sugar and dense carbs added more stress to your life? How does that added stress compare to the feeling of not having sugar and carbs control your food choices and your life?

For those of you on Levels 1 and 2, The 21DSD may have been a huge dietary change. If that's the case, and if you were previously eating bread, cereal, and pasta, then you've essentially been on an elimination diet for three weeks. You need to reintroduce foods slowly (if at all), especially the ones that are highly allergenic, like wheat, dairy, and soy.

To reintroduce foods, here's what you'll need to do:

- The day after your 21DSD ends, choose one food to eat again—most people pick the food they missed the most!

- Eat that food at all three meals along with foods you had included during your detox—meaning that you reintroduce only one potentially problematic food at a time.

- Do not eat that food again for the next two days.

- Note any changes in the following for a full 72 hours after eating the food: mood, energy, appetite, digestive function (like bloating, gas, loose stool, or diarrhea), headaches, inflammation, and mental clarity.

- Your notes will be some of your best guides as to whether you are sensitive to the food you just reintroduced. Food sensitivity reactions can happen immediately, but the onset can also be delayed for up to 72 hours (3 days!).

- I don't recommend ever reintroducing gluten-containing grains like wheat, barley, rye, and spelt, nor do I recommend making pasteurized dairy or unfermented soy products a regular part of your life. These foods are shown to contribute to a myriad of health problems and tend to crowd out much more health-promoting options like vegetables, well-raised meat and eggs, and healthy, naturally occurring fats.

Next, think about how often you used to consume sweetened or carb-rich foods, and then decide whether adding some of those foods back, perhaps once a day instead of at every meal, will be more livable for you on a regular basis. Fruit, for example, is great to enjoy as a dessert or a treat, but most of it isn't included on The 21DSD.

Consider whether you previously ate sweets or dense carbs as rewards, for comfort, or even just by habit. Then ask yourself whether eating them made you feel your best or helped you reach your goals. A lot of people lose weight on The 21DSD, but it's not the primary goal of the program. If you did lose weight, recognize that the bite of sweets here or there that seemed innocent enough before may have been too much for you and your goals. If your primary goal was not weight loss but rather to break unhealthy habits and conquer cravings, think about how eating sweets again will trigger those problems and cause a downward spiral, and then be mindful and conscious when choosing what to eat on a daily basis.

To safely and slowly add some naturally occurring sugars (like fruit) and starches back into your diet, take care to consider the portions and timing of these foods. Fruits should not be eaten alone if you have had problems with blood sugar regulation and cravings. Eat small portions of berries or half a piece of fruit if you're not a very active person, or larger portions if you are more active. Starchy foods are best consumed on days when you are more active, and specifically in the meal following your activity. Otherwise, keep portions of starchy foods to a minimum, and don't allow them to monopolize your plate if weight maintenance is your goal. If you simply want to avoid cravings and you feel okay when you resume eating some starchy foods, then you can enjoy root vegetables, tubers like sweet potatoes, and squash more frequently. Continue to avoid refined foods such as bread, pasta, cereal, and other products made from flour and purchased in packages—these are never healthy options.

The bottom line: After The 21-Day Sugar Detox, a sugar-bender is not recommended. Recall my sugar story: I ate candy when I was hungry after following a sugar-free life for quite some time (this means my blood sugar was already low!). I spiked my blood sugar so high that when it crashed, I nearly passed out. I vowed at that point never to let it happen again. I hope you can learn from my mistake, and from the information outlined above, when choosing how to ease back into your regularly scheduled programming of life and food.

Include estimated quantities/amounts of the foods you eat along with details about those foods. For example, instead of "salad with chicken and balsamic dressing," write "6oz chicken breast, 2c mixed greens, 1/2 avocado, 1/4c shredded carrots, 1/4c cucumber, 1/4c cherry tomatoes, 2 Tbsp EVOO + balsamic vinegar." Using rough estimates is fine, but noting portions will help you as the days continue, since many people undereat on the program. Your journal will help you discover where you can improve on your plan and make it easier to share with others from whom you are seeking support. Below is an example of how to complete your daily log.

DAY # 15

SLEEP TIME
to bed last night _11:30 pm_
woke up today _7:40 am_

SLEEP QUALITY
○ excellent   ○ fair
⊗ good   ○ poor

EXERCISE
time _6:00pm_
type _1 hr CrossFit class_

MOOD & ENERGY
⊗ excellent   ○ fair
○ good   ○ poor

WHAT I ATE FOR...

Breakfast _2 eggs, 1/2 avocado, spinach_

Snack (optional) _1/4 cup almonds 2 oz 21DSD beef jerky_

Lunch _21DSD recipe beef with broccoli – 1 serving_

Dinner _6 oz chicken breast, 2c mixed greens, 1/2 an avocado, 1/4c shredded carrots, 1/4c cucumber, 1/4c cherry tomatoes, 2 Tbsp 21DSD vinaigrette dressing_

Notes _Energy was good today and I felt like I had prepared well for the day – glad I made that beef jerky!_

Use the following page as a format to follow. You can photocopy it or download it as a PDF from balancedbites.com/21DSD.

DAY # ....

SLEEP TIME & QUALITY
to bed last night_____
woke up today_____
○ excellent   ○ fair
○ good   ○ poor

EXERCISE
time   _____
type   _____

MOOD & ENERGY
○ excellent   ○ fair
○ good   ○ poor

WHAT I ATE FOR...
Breakfast_____   Snack (optional)_____
_____   _____
_____   _____
_____   _____

Lunch_____   Dinner_____
_____   _____
_____   _____
_____   _____

Notes_____
_____

DAY # ....

SLEEP TIME & QUALITY
to bed last night_____
woke up today_____
○ excellent   ○ fair
○ good   ○ poor

EXERCISE
time   _____
type   _____

MOOD & ENERGY
○ excellent   ○ fair
○ good   ○ poor

WHAT I ATE FOR...
Breakfast_____   Snack (optional)_____
_____   _____
_____   _____
_____   _____

Lunch_____   Dinner_____
_____   _____
_____   _____
_____   _____

Notes_____
_____

DAY # ....

SLEEP TIME & QUALITY
to bed last night_____
woke up today_____
○ excellent   ○ fair
○ good   ○ poor

EXERCISE
time   _____
type   _____

MOOD & ENERGY
○ excellent   ○ fair
○ good   ○ poor

WHAT I ATE FOR...
Breakfast_____   Snack (optional)_____
_____   _____
_____   _____
_____   _____

Lunch_____   Dinner_____
_____   _____
_____   _____
_____   _____

Notes_____
_____

replacing foods

think ahead to what you will eat in place of some of your favorite
fallbacks while on The 21-Day Sugar Detox

WHAT TO **REPLACE** | WHAT TO **EAT**

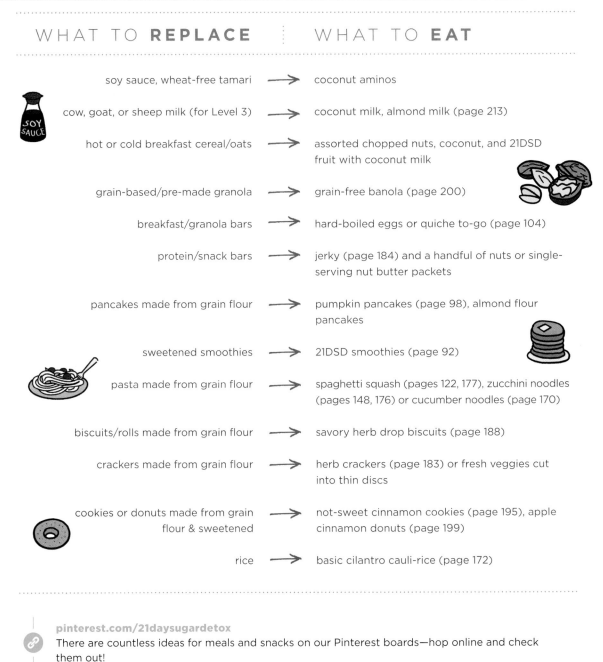

soy sauce, wheat-free tamari	→	coconut aminos
cow, goat, or sheep milk (for Level 3)	→	coconut milk, almond milk (page 213)
hot or cold breakfast cereal/oats	→	assorted chopped nuts, coconut, and 21DSD fruit with coconut milk
grain-based/pre-made granola	→	grain-free banola (page 200)
breakfast/granola bars	→	hard-boiled eggs or quiche to-go (page 104)
protein/snack bars	→	jerky (page 184) and a handful of nuts or single-serving nut butter packets
pancakes made from grain flour	→	pumpkin pancakes (page 98), almond flour pancakes
sweetened smoothies	→	21DSD smoothies (page 92)
pasta made from grain flour	→	spaghetti squash (pages 122, 177), zucchini noodles (pages 148, 176) or cucumber noodles (page 170)
biscuits/rolls made from grain flour	→	savory herb drop biscuits (page 188)
crackers made from grain flour	→	herb crackers (page 183) or fresh veggies cut into thin discs
cookies or donuts made from grain flour & sweetened	→	not-sweet cinnamon cookies (page 195), apple cinnamon donuts (page 199)
rice	→	basic cilantro cauli-rice (page 172)

🔗 pinterest.com/21daysugardetox
There are countless ideas for meals and snacks on our Pinterest boards—hop online and check
them out!

sneaky **sugar synonyms**

all sugar and sweeteners listed here are **out** for The 21-Day Sugar Detox

additional considerations for sweetener choices after The 21-Day Sugar Detox

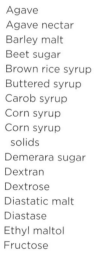

NATURAL SWEETENERS*·················

Brown sugar
Cane juice
Cane juice
  crystals
Cane sugar
Coconut nectar
Coconut sugar/
  crystals

Date sugar
Date syrup
Dates
Fruit juice
Fruit juice
  concentrate
Honey
Maple syrup

Molasses
Palm sugar
Raw sugar
Stevia (green
  leaf or extract)
Turbinado sugar

*Natural sweeteners are the options I recommend using in
very limited quantities *after* your 21DSD.

NATURALLY DERIVED SWEETENERS

Agave
Agave nectar
Barley malt
Beet sugar
Brown rice syrup
Buttered syrup
Carob syrup
Corn syrup
Corn syrup
  solids
Demerara sugar
Dextran
Dextrose
Diastatic malt
Diastase
Ethyl maltol
Fructose

Glucose/
  glucose solids
Golden sugar
Golden syrup
Grape sugar
High-fructose
  corn syrup
Invert sugar
Lactose
Levulose
Light brown
  sugar
Maltitol
Malt syrup
Maltodextrin
Maltose
Mannitol

Muscovado
Refiner's syrup
Sorbitol
Sorghum syrup
Sucrose
Tagatose
  (Tagatesse,
  Nutrilatose)
Treacle
Yellow sugar
Xylitol (or other
  sugar alcohols;
  typically they
  end in "-ose")

ARTIFICIAL SWEETENERS ·················

Acesulfame K/Acesulfame Potassium
  (Sweet One, Sunett)
Aspartame (Equal, NutraSweet)
Saccharine (Sweet'N Low)
Stevia, white/bleached (Truvia, Sun Crystals)
Sucralose (Splenda)

HOW IT'S MADE

The more highly refined a sweetener is, the worse it is for your body. For example, high fructose corn syrup (HFCS) and artificial sweeteners are all very modern, factory made products. Honey, maple syrup, green leaf stevia (dried leaves made into powder), and molasses are all much less processed and have been made for hundreds of years. In the case of honey, almost no processing is necessary. As a result, I vote for raw, organic, local honey as the ideal natural sweetener after your 21DSD.

WHERE IT'S USED

This is a reality check. When you read the ingredients in packaged, processed foods, it becomes obvious that most of them use highly refined, low-quality sweeteners. Food manufacturers even hide sugar in foods that you didn't think were sweet! Many foods that have been made low-fat or non-fat have added sweeteners or artificial sweeteners—avoid these products!

HOW YOUR BODY PROCESSES IT

Here's where the high-fructose corn syrup (HFCS) commercials really get things wrong: Your body actually does not metabolize all sugar the same way. Interestingly enough, sweeteners like HFCS and agave nectar were viewed as better options for diabetics for quite some time because the high fructose content of both requires processing by the liver before the sugar hits your bloodstream. This yielded a seemingly favorable result on blood sugar levels. However, it's now understood that isolated fructose metabolism is a complicated issue and that taxing the liver excessively with such sweeteners can be quite harmful to your health. Fructose is the primary sugar in all fruit. When eating whole fruit, the micronutrients and fiber content of the fruit actually support proper metabolism and assimilation of the fruit sugar. Whole foods for the win! •

dining out

tips and tricks for navigating menus and making healthy choices

AMERICAN FOOD

AVOID: Fried foods, anything breaded, sandwiches, wraps, and pre-mixed dressings.

ENJOY: Bunless or lettuce-wrapped burgers and salads with lemon or vinegar and olive oil.

CHINESE FOOD

AVOID: Unless you know the restaurant well enough to make special requests for no MSG and only sauces without sugar, it's best to avoid Chinese food. Many of the sauces contain hidden sweeteners.

INDIAN FOOD

AVOID: Skip the naan and rice. Ask about flour/gluten in sauces and spice rubs.

ENJOY: Meats and veggies that are grilled or roasted and not drowning in sauces. Tandoori meats are often marinated in yogurt, so they're okay on Levels 1 and 2, but not on Level 3.

ITALIAN FOOD & PIZZA

AVOID: Bread, pasta, and breaded meats. Ask about sauces and preparation of items (meatballs often contain breadcrumbs). There is simply no great way to enjoy a healthy version of pizza while dining out.

ENJOY: Broiled chicken, fish, shrimp, or other protein with red sauce and veggies or salad on the side. If you're craving pizza, make "meatza" at home (recipe on page 126), or make pizza with a cauliflower crust if you are on Level 1 or 2 (which typically include cheese) or an almond meal crust for any level.

JAPANESE FOOD

AVOID: Rice (white and brown) is typically flavored with vinegar, which is okay, but also sugar, which is not. Also avoid anything fried or tempura battered, imitation crab, and most sauces.

ENJOY: Sashimi or broiled fish; just be sure to ask about sauces used and avoid soy sauce.

MEXICAN FOOD

AVOID: Tortilla shells and chips (both corn and flour), beans, and rice (or eat limited portions per Level 1 & 2 guidelines). Vegetarians: Have some beans but go lightly on the rice.

ENJOY: Meat, salsa, and guacamole—often you can ask for these ingredients to be placed over a salad or with vegetables. Ask for raw celery or carrots to dip into guacamole. Ask for a side of vegetables to add to your entrée.

THAI FOOD

AVOID: Sauces that contain peanuts. Also avoid noodles and desserts.

ENJOY: A curry dish or other coconut milk-based dish without rice.

MORE TIPS & TRICKS

smart dining on The 21DSD

Think ahead and don't arrive starving. Eat a small snack of some nuts or nut butter, or even a few bites of avocado or leftover meat before you head out the door.

Preview the restaurant's menu online before you go.

Check out reviews from other diners on a site like Yelp.com or TripAdvisor.com (especially when traveling).

Pass on the bread basket—it'll keep temptation away! Ask for sliced veggies or olives instead.

Either skip the appetizers or opt for a salad starter.

Entrées are easy. While finger food is often breaded, fried, or otherwise carb-loaded, entrées that are made of simpler ingredients can be easy to find.

Look for grilled, broiled, or baked options. These typically aren't breaded, so they'll be safer bets for your detox. But ask the server for details on how things are prepared; they're used to questions! Be polite, but get the answers you need.

Make substitutions. If a meal comes with French fries, bread, or pasta, simply ask that the kitchen either leave it off of the plate or substitute some vegetables instead.

AT PARTIES

Ask the host what they plan on serving so you know what to expect. Bring a dish or two that you know you can enjoy and that will satisfy your hunger. The host will be happy to have the contribution, and you'll be glad to know that you won't be hungry all night if they're serving only foods that you aren't currently eating. ●

fats & oils

cleaning up your diet by using the right fats & oils is essential to improving your health

WHICH TO **EAT**

SATURATED IDEAL FOR HOT USES
PLANT SOURCES *organic, unrefined forms are ideal*

coconut oil
palm oil *from sustainable sources*

ANIMAL SOURCES *pasture-raised/grass-fed & organic sources are ideal*

butter, ghee/clarified butter   schmaltz (chicken fat)
duck fat   tallow
lamb fat
lard

UNSATURATED IDEAL FOR COLD USES
organic, extra-virgin, & cold-pressed forms are ideal

avocado oil   nuts & seeds (including nut &
nut oils (walnut, pecan,   seed butters)
  macadamia)   flaxseed oil (higher in polyunsatu-
olive oil   rated fatty acids, so consume in
sesame oil   extremely limited amounts)

Note: Unsaturated fats—often called oils as listed above—are typically liquid at room temperature and are easily damaged (oxidized) when heat is applied to them. You do not want to consume damaged fats; therefore, cooking in these fats is not recommended.

WHICH TO **DITCH**

SATURATED

Man-made fats are never healthy. Trans fats are particularly harmful.
"Buttery spreads," including oil blends like Earth Balance, Benecol, and
 I Can't Believe It's Not Butter
hydrogenated or partially hydrogenated oils
margarine

UNSATURATED

These oils are highly processed and oxidize easily via one or more of the following: light, air, or heat. Consuming oxidized oils is never healthy.
canola oil (rapeseed oil)   safflower oil
corn oil   soybean oil
grapeseed oil   sunflower oil
rice bran oil   vegetable oil

For more detailed information on the fatty acid profiles of fats & oils, check out my book *Practical Paleo*.

CHOOSING COOKING FATS

listed in order of most stable to least stable for cooking

The fats and oils are ranked below based on the following criteria: 1. how they're made—choose naturally occurring, minimally processed options first; 2. their fatty acid composition— the more saturated they are, the more stable and less likely to be damaged or oxidized they are; 3. smoke point—this tells you how hot is too hot before you will damage the fats, though it should be considered a secondary factor to fatty acid profile.

VERY STABLE—IDEAL FOR COOKING

coconut oil
butter/ghee
cocoa butter
tallow/suet (beef fat)
palm oil *from sustainable sources*
lard/bacon fat (pork fat)
duck fat

MODERATELY STABLE—BEST COLD

avocado oil*
macadamia nut oil*
olive oil*
rice bran oil*

LEAST STABLE—NOT RECOMMENDED

safflower oil**
sesame seed oil**
canola oil**
sunflower oil**
vegetable shortening**
corn oil**
soybean oil**
walnut oil*
grapeseed oil**

*While not recommended for cooking, cold-pressed nut and seed oils that are stored in the refrigerator may be used to finish recipes or after cooking is completed, for flavor.

**These oils are not recommended for consumption, whether hot or cold, but are listed here for your reference, as they are commonly used.

levels & **meal plans**

which level to follow

"Sugar leaves you stranded; I make sure I have the proper amount of protein before I work out." —Evander Holyfield

The 21-Day Sugar Detox has three main levels.

The differences between the levels and modifications for the various tracks, while minor at first glance, translate into some very different food choices on a daily basis. In order to determine which level you should follow, as well as any possible modifications you may want to make, complete this short self-quiz.

SELF-QUIZ

Select the answer that **best** describes you.

1. Are you new to The 21-Day Sugar Detox?
   a) yes
   b) no, I have completed it once
   c) no, I have completed it two or more times

2. I currently eat:
   a) bread, pasta, and other foods made from whole grain or other types of grain flour (wheat, teff, spelt, kamut, rye, etc.)
   b) bread, pasta, and other foods made from gluten-free grain flours
   c) a grain-free, Paleo, or primal type of diet

3. I currently eat:
   a) fat-free dairy products
   b) low-fat dairy products
   c) full-fat dairy products or no dairy

4. I feel that my sugar and carb cravings are:
   a) *so* strong that I'm admittedly fearful of how this detox will go for me
   b) pretty darned strong—that's why I'm reading this!
   c) not terrible, but certainly not under control the way I think they should be

5. I:
   a) am currently following a pescetarian diet—I eat seafood, eggs, and dairy, but not meat
   b) am currently pregnant or nursing one or more children
   c) live a very active lifestyle, work at a physically demanding job, or participate in high-intensity physical activity or exercise regularly
   d) have been diagnosed with an autoimmune condition
   e) none of the above

Results

QUESTIONS #1–4

Determines which level is right for you.

- If you answered mostly "a," then select **Level 1.**
- If you answered mostly "b," then select **Level 2.**
- If you answered mostly "c," then select **Level 3.**

QUESTION #5

Determines the modifications, if any, to the level you determined was right for you based on your answers to questions #1-4.

- If you answered "a," then follow the Pescetarian modifications on page 73 (for Level 1) or page 81 (for Level 2).
- If you answered "b" or "c," then follow the Energy modifications on page 72 (for Level 1), page 80 (for Level 2), or page 88 (for Level 3).
- If you answered "d," then follow the Autoimmune modifications on page 89.
- If you answered "e," then simply follow the level that is right for you.

While Level 1 is the most lenient plan and Level 3 is the strictest, Level 1 will likely be your best bet if dietary changes are a new endeavor for you. That said, the level you tackle is *absolutely your choice.* You may find that Level 1 is a great choice for your first time through, and that returning to complete the program at Level 2, then Level 3 later on will be quite effective and present different challenges and results.

THE MODIFICATIONS

The Pescetarian, Energy, and Autoimmune modifications have been created to enhance your experience if you fall into one of those categories for nutritional needs. It's important that you include the recommended modifications, as you will likely struggle with more severe detox symptoms. Each track has some specifications that are not necessarily aligned with every level. For example, the Pescetarian modifications are not appropriate in combination with Level 3 food choices since that level omits many foods that pescetarians will need to rely on for nutrition.

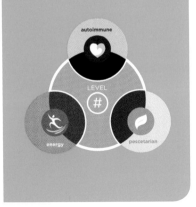

• DON'T BE A HERO! •
An important note about selecting a level and following modifications

The levels and modifications were created and refined after thousands of people completed the program. Completing a higher level just to challenge yourself more is not necessarily going to yield a better result.

You can always come back for another round of The 21DSD at a different level or using different modifications after you complete this one, but use this guide to best determine where to start each time! ●

Is it a "Yes" food?

While you follow the guidelines and Yes/No Foods Lists outlined in the following pages, you may encounter foods that are not listed, or you may be slightly confused about whether a particular food is included in or excluded from the program. Read the Yes/No Foods List for your level thoroughly, then follow these basic principles of The 21DSD to direct your choices and help you figure out whether or not you should eat the food in question.

- **Added sweeteners are not allowed.** The only way to enjoy a somewhat sweet taste is to use the included fruits in the limited portions as outlined in your Yes/No Foods List. If an added sweetener is included in the ingredients list of a packaged item you want to eat (see page 59 for Sneaky Sugar Synonyms to find hidden sweeteners), it is not allowed. See the FAQ about bacon on page 49 for the one exception to this rule. Note that some foods on your Yes list, such as full-fat dairy on Levels 1 and 2, contain natural sugars, and these are okay.

- **If it tastes sweet and it isn't included on the Yes or Limit foods list for your level, it's not allowed.** Some herbal teas taste sweet naturally, and these are allowed. If an item tastes sweet and you aren't sure about it, leave it out.

- **Grain flours are not allowed.** This means you will not eat any foods made from whole-grain or refined-grain flours (wheat, spelt, and quinoa flours, for example). The only flours allowed are those made from nuts, seeds, coconut, or some limited starches (like tapioca flour when used as a thickening agent in sauces).

- **When in doubt, leave it out.** If you find it difficult to make a judgment call about a particular food on your own, login to the forums at balancedbites.com/21DSD to ask your question and get more answers and support.

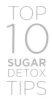

TOP
10
SUGAR
DETOX
TIPS

1. SLEEP. If you're not getting enough sleep, you're setting yourself up for a full day's worth of cravings.

2. DRINK WATER. Stay hydrated to be sure that when you are feeling hungry, it's not actually thirst kicking in.

3. BE PREPARED. Having the right foods on hand will get you through the day so that you can do your best to avoid cravings, but will have good food available if they hit.

4. ENLIST A FRIEND. Or coworker, or family member...you get the idea. Completing this challenge with the support of someone you spend time with daily can help tons.

5. LEARN TO LOVE HERBAL TEA. You can drink herbal tea (caffeine-free) to your heart's content. It often feels like a treat, so you won't feel deprived if you have a craving.

6. PROTEIN FIRST, THEN FAT, THEN VEGGIES. That's how you build a plate, whether it's a meal or a snack.

7. TURN MEALS INTO SNACKS. Prepare just a little bit extra when you make a meal, and stash leftovers in a container for a snack if you need it. A snack doesn't need to be "snack food."

8. TAKE A WALK. When you feel like you want a sweet treat, a distraction or some physical activity can often get your mind refocused.

9. REDUCE CAFFEINE. Caffeine encourages your body to crave sugar. If you're struggling, work on reducing your caffeine intake over the first week.

10. RELAX! Stressing about the detox will only make you crave more sugar!

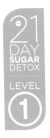

level 1

notes for level 1 that explain its differences from the other levels

While completing The 21-Day Sugar Detox at Level 1, you may choose to follow this meal plan to the letter, follow parts of it to suit your needs and tastes, or simply follow your Yes/No Foods List on page 70-71 along with these general notes.

The following foods are optional to include with meals or snacks; you can leave them out if you choose on some days. *Optional meal plan items appear in italics.*

WHOLE GRAINS & LEGUMES
up to 1/2 cup total per day, cooked

Only gluten-free grains are included in this program.

- amaranth
- arrowroot
- beans: black, fava, navy, pinto, red
- buckwheat
- garbanzo beans (chickpeas)
- lentils
- millet
- quinoa
- rice (white, brown, wild)
- sorghum
- tapioca

Note that foods made *from* the included whole grains (for instance, brown rice pasta and whole-grain cereals) are *not* approved.

If you are following the meal plan provided here, I have added your 1/2 cup per day of grains or legumes to meals in the plan based on the cuisine types and flavor combinations.

If you are not following the meal plan specifically, you will need to add your 1/2 cup serving where you see fit. If you plan on cooking from the recipes in this book, they are approved for *all* levels and do not include grains or legumes.

Feel free to adjust the time of day you include your portion. For example, if rice is planned at lunch but you generally feel better including your additional carbs at dinner, you can absolutely do that. In general, I find that including carbs later in the day leads to better sleep and more even blood sugar levels throughout the day.

FULL-FAT DAIRY *no specific portion limits*
Non-fat and low-fat dairy products are not allowed.

- cheese, cream cheese, cottage cheese
- whole milk, heavy cream, half & half
- plain full-fat yogurt or kefir
- sour cream

You may choose to include full-fat dairy in your daily meal plan, or just occasionally. There are some suggestions of where you may add it within the plan that follows. Choose local, grass-fed, and non-homogenized varieties whenever possible. Organic is recommended if you are unable to find grass-fed dairy.

BALANCEDBITES.COM/21DSD
Printable shopping lists are available online.

level 1

DAY	BREAKFAST	LUNCH	DINNER	SNACK
1 ● ● ▲ ■	buffalo chicken egg muffins (100), steamed spinach, avocado	salmon salad with capers & tomato (154), leafy greens salad or wraps	mini mexi-meatloaves (118), creamy herb mashed cauliflower (178) or *1/2 cup rice* or **black beans**	simple beef jerky (184) + Choice of nut mix (192)
2 ● ● ■ ▲	*leftover* buffalo chicken egg muffins, steamed spinach, avocado	*leftover* mini mexi-meatloaves, basic cilantro cauli-rice (172) or *1/2 cup rice* or **black beans**	broiled salmon with caper & olive tapenade (146), mixed greens salad	*leftover* simple beef jerky + *leftover* nut mix
3 ♦ ▲ ●	green apple breakfast sausage (94), raw carrot sticks, raw almonds	*leftover* broiled salmon, simple spinach & garlic soup (162) or *1/2 cup quinoa*, mixed greens with vinaigrette (218)	mustard-glazed chicken thighs (114), golden beets with crispy herbs (180) or green vegetable*	hard-boiled egg + baked kale chips (190)
4 ♦ ● ♦	*leftover* green apple breakfast sausage, raw carrot sticks, raw almonds or walnuts	*leftover* mustard-glazed chicken thighs, *leftover* golden beets with crispy herbs or green vegetable*	asian-style meatballs (138), fresh cabbage & bok choy slaw (171), no-miso soup (164), *1/2 cup rice*	21DSD-friendly fruit + nut butter or **full-fat yogurt**
5 ♦ ♦ ■	bacon & root veggie hash (95), 2 eggs any style or 3oz protein of choice	*leftover* asian-style meatballs, *leftover* fresh cabbage & bok choy slaw, *1/2 cup brown rice*	shepherd's pie (134), green salad with dressing of choice (216-218)	grain-free banola (200) **+ milk, coconut milk,** or **full-fat yogurt**
6 ♦ ■ ▲	*leftover* bacon & root veggie hash, 2 eggs any style or 3oz protein of choice	*leftover* shepherd's pie, green salad with dressing of choice (216-218)	shrimp pad thai (148), *1/2 cup brown rice sautéed with coconut aminos*	*leftover* grain-free banola **+ milk, coconut milk,** or **full-fat yogurt**
7 ▲ ● ▲ ♦	*leftover* shrimp pad thai	perfectly grilled chicken breast (106), broccoli & bacon salad with creamy balsamic vinaigrette (169)	seafood & chorizo paella (142), *mix 1/2 cup cooked brown rice into the cauli-rice per serving*	simple beef jerky (184) + cinnilla nut mix (192)

KEY
- ● Eggs
- ● Poultry
- ♦ Pork
- ■ Lamb
- ■ Beef/Bison
- ▲ Seafood

NOTES
*   choose any green vegetable from your Yes foods list on page 70
**   add a starchy vegetable if you are following modifications that direct you to do so
Bold italicized items are optional—you can add them or leave them out.
Icons denote the main protein source in meals for your planning purposes. Snacks are optional.

level 1

DAY	BREAKFAST	LUNCH	DINNER	SNACK
8 ● ● ■	tomato-basil quiche with bacon & spinach (104)	*leftover* perfectly grilled chicken breast, lemon & garlic noodles with olives (176)	ginger-garlic beef & broccoli (130), basic cilantro cauli-rice (172) or *1/2 cup brown rice*	*leftover* simple beef jerky + *leftover* cinnilla nut mix (192)
9 ● ■ ◆	*leftover* tomato-basil quiche with bacon & spinach	*leftover* ginger-garlic beef & broccoli, *leftover* basic cilantro cauli-rice	double pork tenderloin (140), green apple & fennel salad (168), *1/2 cup quinoa*	21DSD-friendly fruit + nut butter or *full-fat yogurt*
10 ● ◆ ▲	lemon chicken with capers & chives (109), raw carrot sticks or steamed vegetables*	*leftover* double pork tenderloin, green salad with dressing of choice (216-218)	lemon sole with almonds & thyme (145), roasted cauliflower soup (160), *1/2 cup quinoa*	21DSD-friendly fruit + nut butter or *full-fat yogurt*
11 ● ▲ ■	*leftover* lemon chicken with capers & chives, raw carrot sticks or steamed vegetables*	tuna salad wraps (152), *leftover* roasted cauliflower soup or green vegetable*	greek-style meatballs & salad (129), greek tomato & cucumber salad (175), *1/2 cup rice*	grain-free banola (200) *+ milk, coconut milk,* or *full-fat yogurt*
12 ◆ ■ ●	green apple breakfast sausage (94), raw carrot sticks or other vegetables*	*leftover* greek-style meatballs & salad	hot & sweet ginger-garlic chicken (116), cucumber cold noodle salad (170), *1/2 cup brown rice*	*leftover* grain-free banola *+ milk, coconut milk,* or *full-fat yogurt*
13 ◆ ● ■	*leftover* breakfast sausage, raw carrot sticks, raw almonds or walnuts	*leftover* hot & sweet ginger-garlic chicken, green vegetable*, *1/2 cup brown rice*	spaghetti squash bolognese (122), green salad	simple beef jerky (184) + choice of nut mix (192)
14 ● ■ ◆	veggie pancakes (97), 3oz protein of choice	*leftover* spaghetti squash bolognese, green salad	cinnamon grilled pork chops (141), crumb-topped brussels sprouts (181), *1/2 cup quinoa*	*leftover* simple beef jerky + *leftover* nut mix

KEY
- ● Eggs
- ● Poultry
- ◆ Pork
- ■ Lamb
- ■ Beef/Bison
- ▲ Seafood

NOTES

*   choose any green vegetable from your Yes foods list on page 70

**   add a starchy vegetable if you are following modifications that direct you to do so

Bold italicized items are optional—you can add them or leave them out.

Icons denote the main protein source in meals for your planning purposes. Snacks are optional.

68   THE 21-DAY SUGAR DETOX • DIANE SANFILIPPO

level 1

DAY	BREAKFAST	LUNCH	DINNER	SNACK
15 ● ◆ ▲	carrot pumpkin spice muffins (103), 2 eggs any style, or 3oz protein of choice	*leftover* cinnamon grilled pork chops, *leftover* crumb-topped brussels sprouts, *1/2 cup quinoa*	buffalo shrimp lettuce cups (156), basic 4 guacamole (185), jicama fresh "fries" (174)	21DSD-friendly fruit + nut butter or *full-fat yogurt*
16 ● ● ■ ◆	*leftover* carrot pumpkin spice muffins, 2 eggs any style or 3oz protein of choice	smoky chicken tortilla-less soup (158), *leftover* basic 4 guacamole, *1/2 cup rice*	stovetop lamb & chorizo chili (136), cocoa-chili roasted cauliflower (179)	21DSD-friendly fruit + nut butter or *full-fat yogurt*
17 ▲ ■ ◆ ●	rosemary salmon with cabbage (96)	*leftover* stovetop lamb & chorizo chili, *leftover* cocoa-chili roasted cauliflower	chicken with artichokes & olives (110), *1/2 cup garbanzo beans,* lemon & garlic noodles with olives (176)	grain-free banola (200) *+ milk, coconut milk,* or *full-fat yogurt*
18 ● ■	smoothie of choice (92-93) with 2 eggs any style or 3oz protein of choice	*leftover* chicken with artichokes & olives, *1/2 cup garbanzo beans,* *leftover* lemon & garlic noodles with olives	meatza two-ways (126), pesto spaghetti squash (177)	*leftover* grain-free banola *+ milk, coconut milk,* or *full-fat yogurt*
19 ■ ●	smoothie of choice (92-93) with 2 eggs any style or 3oz protein of choice	[make ahead] italian-style stuffed bell peppers (124)	chicken with tri-color peppers (108), basic cilantro cauli-rice (172) or *1/2 cup rice*	simple beef jerky (184) + choice of nut mix (192)
20 ● ▲	savory herb drop biscuits (188), 3oz protein of choice, veggies of choice*	[make ahead] rainbow collard wraps with herb almond "cheese" spread (150)	spicy sesame-lime salmon (144), cucumber cold noodle salad (170), *1/2 cup rice* or *quinoa*	*leftover* simple beef jerky + *leftover* nut mix
21 ● ● ■	tomato-basil quiche with bacon & spinach (104)	*perfectly grilled chicken breast (106), lemon & garlic noodles with olives (176), *1/2 cup red beans*	jalapeño bacon burgers (120) with veggie pancakes (97)	21DSD-friendly fruit + nut butter or *full-fat yogurt*

KEY
- ● Eggs
- ● Poultry
- ◆ Pork
- ■ Lamb
- ■ Beef/Bison
- ▲ Seafood

NOTES

*   choose any green vegetable from your Yes foods list on page 70

**   add a starchy vegetable if you are following modifications that direct you to do so

***Bold italicized items** are optional—you can add them or leave them out.*

Icons denote the main protein source in meals for your planning purposes. Snacks are optional.

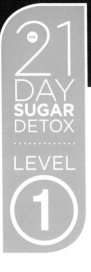

THE 21 DAY SUGAR DETOX

LEVEL 1

**DON'T SEE THE
FOOD YOU WANT TO
EAT ON THE LIST?**

Review "Is it a Yes food?"
on page 65.

MODIFICATIONS

If you are following the
Energy or Pescetarian
track, see the meal plan
modifications on pages
72-73 for additional notes.

YES FOODS *eat plenty of these foods for 21 days*

MEAT, FISH, & EGGS
including but not limited to:
ALL meats, including deli
and cured meats like ba-
con, pancetta, prosciutto,
etc. (see page 224 for the
best brands & ingredients
to avoid)
ALL seafood
Eggs

VEGETABLES
Artichokes/sunchokes
Asparagus
Broccoli
Brussels sprouts
Cabbage
Carrots
Cauliflower
Celery/celery root
Chard
Collards
Cucumber
Eggplant
Garlic
Ginger
Green beans
Horseradish
Jicama
Kale
Leeks
Lettuce, *all leafy greens*
Mushrooms
Onions
Parsnips
Peppers, *all varieties*
Radicchio
Radishes
Rutabaga
Snow/snap peas
Spaghetti squash
Spinach
Tomato
Turnips
Yellow squash
Zucchini

FRUIT
*review the Limit foods for more
fruit choices!*
Lemon
Lime

NUTS/SEEDS
whole, flour, or butters
Almonds
Brazil nuts
Cocoa/cacao (100%), nibs
Chia seeds
Coconut, *all unsweetened
forms are okay—coconut
sugar is a NO*
Filberts (hazelnuts)
Flax seeds
Hemp seeds
Macadamias
Pecans
Pistachios
Pumpkin seeds
Sunflower seeds
Sesame seeds, tahini
Walnuts

FATS & OILS
review the guide on page 61
Animal fats
Butter, ghee, clarified
butter
Avocados, avocado oil
Coconut oil
Flax oil
Olives, olive oil
Sesame oil

DAIRY
full-fat only!
Cheese, cream cheese, cot-
tage cheese
Milk, whole only
Half & half
Heavy cream
Sour cream
Yogurt/kefir, plain

BEVERAGES
Almond milk, unsweetened/
homemade (page 213)
Coconut milk, coconut
cream, full-fat
Coffee, espresso
Mineral water
Seltzer, club soda
Teas: herbal, green, black,
white, etc., unsweetened
Water

CONDIMENTS/MISC.
Broth, homemade only
(recipe on page 212)
Coconut aminos
21DSD Ketchup (recipe on
page 214)
*no store-bought ketchups
are allowed*
Extracts:
vanilla, almond, etc., and
vanilla bean
Hummus made using
cauliflower
Healthy Homemade Mayon-
naise (recipe on page 211)
*do your best to avoid
others*
Mustard, gluten-free
varieties
Nutritional/Brewer's yeast
(Lewis Labs brand)
Salad dressings,
homemade
Spices & herbs:
all are OK; check pre-
mixed blends for hidden
ingredients
Vinegars:
apple cider, balsamic,
distilled, red wine, sherry,
white

SUPPLEMENTS
Protein powder, 100% pure
with NO other ingredients
(e.g., 100% whey, egg
white, or hemp)
Fermented cod liver oil,
with or without flavor
(one exception to the no-
sweetener rule!)
Pure vitamin or mineral
supplements

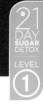

LIMIT FOODS *these are Yes foods with portion size limits*

VEGETABLES & STARCHES
1 cup serving per day is allowed

Acorn squash
Beets
Butternut squash
Green peas
Pumpkin
Winter squash (assorted)

FRUIT
1 piece per day is allowed

Bananas, green-tipped/
  not quite ripe only
Grapefruit
Green/Granny Smith
  apples

GRAINS/LEGUMES
*1/2 cup serving per day
(cooked) is allowed of whole
forms only—NO FLOURS*

Amaranth
Arrowroot
Beans: black, fava,
  garbanzo (chickpeas),
  navy, pinto, red
Buckwheat
Lentils
Millet
Quinoa
Rice (brown, white, wild)
Sorghum

BEVERAGES
1 cup total per day is allowed

Coconut juice, coconut
  water:
  no added sweeteners
Kombucha, home-
  brewed or store-bought
  (see FAQs on pages 46
  and 51, and recom-
  mended brands on
  page 224)

NO FOODS *do not eat these foods for 21 days*

REFINED CARBOHYDRATES
Bagels
Bread
Breadsticks
Brownies
Cake
Candy
Cereal/granola
Chips
Cookies
Couscous
Crackers
Croissants
Cupcakes
Muffins
Oats
Orzo
Pasta
Pastries
Pita
Pizza
Popcorn
Rice cakes
Rolls
Tortillas, tortilla chips

VEGETABLES & STARCHES
Cassava
Corn, polenta, grits
Plantains
Soybeans/edamame
Sweet potatoes/yams
Tapioca, whole & flour
Taro

FRUITS
*review the Yes and Limit foods
lists for the included fruits*
Fresh & dried

GRAINS/LEGUMES
Barley
Kamut
Rye
Soybeans/edamame
  (including miso, natto,
  tempeh, tofu, and soy
  sauce)
Spelt
Wheat
Flours made from grains
  or beans (chickpeas,
  lentils, etc.)

NUTS/NUT BUTTERS
Cashew
Peanut

SWEETENERS OF ANY KIND
None are allowed! See
page 59 for a complete
list to help you identify
hidden sweeteners.

ANYTHING "DIET," SUGAR-FREE, OR ARTIFICIALLY SWEETENED
This means no gum
either!

SUPPLEMENTS
Anything that includes
  sugar, sweeteners, or
  sugar alcohols (xylitol,
  for example)
Shakeology and other
  similar blends
Supplements that con-
  tain soy, corn, or wheat

BEVERAGES
All alcohol
Coffee "drinks" or shakes,
  pre-sweetened
Juice
Milk: skim, non-fat, 1%,
  2%, soy/rice/oat
Soda (regular & diet)
Sweet-tasting drinks
  (besides herbal teas)
Protein powders that
  have more than one
  ingredient (see Yes food
  supplements)

CONDIMENTS/MISC.
Broth/stock in a box/can
Hummus, made from
  garbanzo beans
Ketchup, store-bought
Mayonnaise, store-bought
Salad dressings, pre-
  made/store-bought
Soy sauce, tamari

level 1 energy

additional notes for those who need more carbohydrates

THESE MODIFICATIONS MAY BE RIGHT FOR YOU IF YOU

· live a very active lifestyle or work at a physically demanding job
· participate in high-intensity physical activity or exercise regularly (for example, interval training, CrossFit-style workouts, endurance athletics, or cardio/aerobic activity at moderate to high intensity for more than 20 minutes at a time; yoga alone doesn't typically require these modifications)
· are pregnant or nursing

With the Energy modifications, your portion of whole grains or legumes will increase. You will also need to add starchy carbohydrate vegetables to your meal plan that are considered No foods for those who do not fit the modification requirements listed above.

WHOLE GRAINS & LEGUMES
include up to 1 cup total per day, cooked
As noted under the Limit foods on your Yes/No Foods List.

STARCHY CARBOHYDRATE VEGETABLES
amount varies based on your activity level and energy requirements; see page 221 for a list of these foods
Add 30–50 grams of carbohydrates to a *minimum* of one meal per day, especially after exercise. This means 1/2 to 1 cup of mashed sweet potato, for example. You should also use the one piece of fruit per day included for all Level 1 detoxers to reach this carbohydrate goal.

If you train very hard (at high intensity, or more than once a day), you may need to make this modification for *each instance* of exercise—meaning more than one meal or snack will include up to this amount of dense carbohydrates.

You may adjust what time of day you include your extra carbs. For example, if sweet potato is listed at lunch but you generally feel better including your additional carbs at dinner, you can absolutely do that. In general, adding more carbs later in the day or after activity tends to replenish your fuel better. *This is a highly variable element in your meal planning, and tracking your own energy levels is the best way to decide when to time your extra carbs.*

RECOMMENDED CARBS PER DAY
Moderately active: 75–150 grams
Highly active: 100–200+ grams
Pregnant/nursing: 100+ grams
These are estimates. If you find that you need more carbs to maintain activity, adjust to your needs.

If you are pregnant or nursing one or more children, add these carbohydrate sources as you see fit. Do not limit them assuming it will lead to better results. The goal of this program is a healthy body and a healthy baby, and limiting these foods further is absolutely not necessary! If you find that your milk supply is low or you feel more fatigued than usual, increase your intake of more carbohydrate-dense foods as outlined here.

*additional notes for those who eat
seafood, eggs, and dairy, but not meat*

THESE MODIFICATIONS MAY BE RIGHT FOR YOU IF YOU
· follow a pescetarian diet

With the Pescetarian modifications, your portion of whole grains or legumes will increase. You will also need to add starchy carbohydrate vegetables to your meal plan that are considered No foods for those who do not fit the modification requirements listed above.

WHOLE GRAINS & LEGUMES
you may include up to 1 cup per day total, cooked
As noted under the Limit foods on your Yes/No Foods List. It is not required that you eat the approved grains or legumes every day if you are eating sufficient amounts of other protein and carb sources.

STARCHY CARBOHYDRATE VEGETABLES
you may include up to 2 cups per day; see page 221 for a list of these foods

FULL-FAT DAIRY *no specific portion limits*
You may want to add some high-quality dairy to meals for additional protein and fat. Choose local, grass-fed, and non-homogenized varieties whenever possible. Organic is recommended if you are unable to find grass-fed dairy.

EXTRA FATS
add extra fat portions to meals and snacks
For example:
· add a whole avocado to a meal instead of a half
· add 1/4 cup nuts and/or dressing to a salad instead of 2 tablespoons
· make good use of full-fat dairy products for fat and protein if you tolerate dairy well (tolerating dairy means that you don't experience symptoms such as gas, bloating, digestive distress, acne, eczema, or congestion when you eat it)

SEAFOOD
make seafood your protein source in at least one meal per day, ideally two

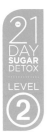

level 2

notes for level 2 that explain its differences from the other levels

While completing The 21-Day Sugar Detox at Level 2, you may choose to follow this meal plan to the letter, follow parts of it to suit your needs or tastes, or simply follow your Yes/No Foods List on pages 78-79 along with these general notes.

The following foods are optional to include with meals or snacks; you can leave them out if you choose on some days. *Optional meal plan items appear in italics.*

FULL-FAT DAIRY
no specific portion limits

Non-fat or low-fat dairy products are not allowed.

· cheese, cream cheese, cottage cheese
· whole milk, heavy cream, half & half
· plain full-fat yogurt or kefir
· sour cream

You may choose to include full-fat dairy in your daily meal plan, or just occasionally. There are some suggestions of where you may add it within the plan that follows. Choose local, grass-fed, and non-homogenized varieties whenever possible. Organic is recommended if you are unable to find grass-fed dairy.

BALANCEDBITES.COM/21DSD
Printable shopping lists are available online.

DAY	BREAKFAST	LUNCH	DINNER	SNACK
1 ● ● ▲ ■	buffalo chicken egg muffins (100), steamed spinach, avocado	salmon salad with capers & tomato (154), leafy greens salad or wraps	mini mexi-meatloaves (118), creamy herb mashed cauliflower, **use cilantro** (178)	simple beef jerky (184) + choice of nut mix (192)
2 ● ● ■ ▲	*leftover* buffalo chicken egg muffins, steamed spinach, avocado	*leftover* mini mexi-meatloaves, basic cilantro cauli-rice (172)	broiled salmon with caper & olive tapenade (146), mixed greens salad	*leftover* simple beef jerky + *leftover* nut mix
3 ♦ ▲ ●	green apple breakfast sausage (94), raw carrot sticks, raw almonds	*leftover* broiled salmon, simple spinach & garlic soup (162) or mixed greens with balsamic vinaigrette dressing (218)	mustard-glazed chicken thighs (114), golden beets with crispy herbs (180) or green vegetable*	hard-boiled egg + baked kale chips (190)
4 ♦ ● ♦	*leftover* green apple breakfast sausage, raw carrot sticks, raw almonds or walnuts	*leftover* mustard-glazed chicken thighs, *leftover* golden beets with crispy herbs or green vegetable*	asian-style meatballs (138), fresh cabbage & bok choy slaw (171), no-miso soup (164)	21DSD-friendly fruit + nut butter or **full-fat yogurt**
5 ♦ ♦ ■	bacon & root veggie hash (95), 2 eggs any style or 3oz protein of choice	*leftover* asian-style meatballs, *leftover* fresh cabbage & bok choy slaw	shepherd's pie (134), green salad with dressing of choice (216-218)	grain-free banola (200) *+ milk, coconut milk, or full-fat yogurt*
6 ♦ ■ ▲	*leftover* bacon & root veggie hash, 2 eggs any style or 3oz protein of choice	*leftover* shepherd's pie, green salad with dressing of choice (216-218)	shrimp pad thai (148)	*leftover* grain-free banola *+ milk, coconut milk, or full-fat yogurt*
7 ▲ ● ▲ ♦	*leftover* shrimp pad thai	perfectly grilled chicken breast (106), broccoli & bacon salad with creamy balsamic dressing (169)	seafood & chorizo paella (142)	simple beef jerky (184) + cinnilla nut mix (192)

KEY
- ● Eggs
- ● Poultry
- ♦ Pork
- ■ Lamb
- ■ Beef/Bison
- ▲ Seafood

NOTES
*   choose any green vegetable from your Yes foods list on page 78
**   add a starchy vegetable if you are following modifications that direct you to do so
Bold italicized items are optional—you can add them or leave them out.
Icons denote the main protein source in meals for your planning purposes. Snacks are optional.

level 2

DAY	BREAKFAST	LUNCH	DINNER	SNACK
8 ● ● ■	tomato-basil quiche with bacon & spinach (104)	*leftover* perfectly grilled chicken breast, lemon & garlic noodles with olives (176)	ginger-garlic beef & broccoli (130), basic cilantro cauli-rice (172)	*leftover* simple beef jerky + *leftover* cinnilla nut mix
9 ● ■ ◆	*leftover* tomato-basil quiche with bacon & spinach	*leftover* ginger-garlic beef & broccoli, *leftover* basic cilantro cauli-rice	double pork tenderloin (140), green apple & fennel salad (168)	21DSD-friendly fruit + nut butter or **full-fat yogurt**
10 ● ◆ ▲	lemon chicken with capers & chives (109), raw carrot sticks or steamed vegetables*	*leftover* double pork tenderloin, green salad with dressing of choice (216-218)	lemon sole with almonds & thyme (145), roasted cauliflower soup (160)	21DSD-friendly fruit + nut butter or **full-fat yogurt**
11 ● ▲ ■	*leftover* lemon chicken with capers & chives, raw carrot sticks or steamed vegetables*	tuna salad wraps (152), *leftover* roasted cauliflower soup or green vegetable*	greek-style meatballs & salad (129), greek tomato & cucumber salad (175)	grain-free banola (200) **+ milk, coconut milk,** or **full-fat yogurt**
12 ◆ ■ ●	green apple breakfast sausage (94), raw carrot sticks or other vegetables*	*leftover* greek-style meatballs & salad	hot & sweet ginger-garlic chicken (116), cucumber cold noodle salad (170)	*leftover* grain-free banola **+ milk, coconut milk,** or **full-fat yogurt**
13 ◆ ● ■	*leftover* green apple breakfast sausage, raw carrot sticks, raw almonds or walnuts	*leftover* hot & sweet ginger-garlic chicken, green vegetable*	spaghetti squash bolognese (122), green salad	simple beef jerky (184) + choice of nut mix (192)
14 ● ■ ◆	veggie pancakes (97), 3oz protein of choice	*leftover* spaghetti squash bolognese, green salad	cinnamon grilled pork chops (141), crumb-topped brussels sprouts (181)	*leftover* simple beef jerky + *leftover* nut mix

KEY
- ● Eggs
- ● Poultry
- ◆ Pork
- ■ Lamb
- ■ Beef/Bison
- ▲ Seafood

NOTES

*   choose any green vegetable from your Yes foods list on page 78

**   add a starchy vegetable if you are following modifications that direct you to do so

Bold italicized items are optional—you can add them or leave them out.

Icons denote the main protein source in meals for your planning purposes. Snacks are optional.

level 2

DAY	BREAKFAST	LUNCH	DINNER	SNACK
15 ● ◆ ▲	carrot pumpkin spice muffins (103), 2 eggs any style or 3oz protein of choice	*leftover* cinnamon grilled pork chops, *leftover* crumb-topped brussels sprouts	buffalo shrimp lettuce cups (156), basic 4 guacamole (185), jicama fresh "fries" (174)	21DSD-friendly fruit + nut butter or ***full-fat yogurt***
16 ● ● ■ ◆	*leftover* carrot pumpkin spice muffins, 2 eggs any style or 3oz protein of choice	smoky chicken tortilla-less soup (158), *leftover* basic 4 guacamole	stovetop lamb & chorizo chili (136), cocoa-chili roasted cauliflower (179)	21DSD-friendly fruit + nut butter or ***full-fat yogurt***
17 ▲ ■ ◆ ●	rosemary salmon with cabbage (96)	*leftover* stovetop lamb & chorizo chili, *leftover* cocoa-chili roasted cauliflower	chicken with artichokes & olives (110), lemon & garlic noodles with olives (176)	grain-free banola (200) ***+ milk, coconut milk,*** or ***full-fat yogurt***
18 ● ■	smoothie of choice (92-93) with 2 eggs any style or 3oz protein of choice	*leftover* chicken with artichokes & olives, *leftover* lemon & garlic noodles with olives	meatza two-ways (126), pesto spaghetti squash (177)	*leftover* grain-free banola ***+ milk, coconut milk,*** or ***full-fat yogurt***
19 ■ ●	smoothie of choice (92-93) with 2 eggs any style or 3oz protein of choice	[make ahead] italian-style stuffed bell peppers (124)	chicken with tri-color peppers (108), basic cilantro cauli-rice (172)	simple beef jerky (184) + cinnilla nut mix (192)
20 ● ▲	savory herb drop biscuits (188), 3oz protein of choice, green vegetable*	[make ahead] rainbow collard wraps with herb almond "cheese" spread (150)	spicy sesame-lime salmon (144), cucumber cold noodle salad (170)	*leftover* simple beef jerky + *leftover* cinnilla nut mix
21 ● ● ■	tomato-basil quiche with bacon & spinach (104)	perfectly grilled chicken breast (106), lemon & garlic noodles with olives (176)	jalapeño bacon burgers (120) with veggie pancakes (97)	21DSD-friendly fruit + nut butter or ***full-fat yogurt***

KEY
- ● Eggs
- ● Poultry
- ◆ Pork
- ■ Lamb
- ■ Beef/Bison
- ▲ Seafood

NOTES

*   choose any green vegetable from your Yes foods list on page 78

**   add a starchy vegetable if you are following modifications that direct you to do so

Bold italicized items are optional—you can add them or leave them out.

Icons denote the main protein source in meals for your planning purposes. Snacks are optional.

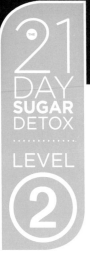

21 DAY SUGAR DETOX

LEVEL 2

DON'T SEE THE FOOD YOU WANT TO EAT ON THE LIST?

Review "Is it a Yes food?" on page 65.

MODIFICATIONS

If you are following the Energy or Pescetarian track, see the meal plan modifications on pages 80-81 for additional notes.

YES FOODS *eat plenty of these foods for 21 days*

MEAT, FISH, & EGGS
including but not limited to:
ALL meats, including deli and cured meats like bacon, pancetta, prosciutto, etc. (see page 224 for the best brands & ingredients to avoid)
ALL seafood
Eggs

VEGETABLES
Artichokes/sunchokes
Asparagus
Broccoli
Brussels sprouts
Cabbage
Carrots
Cauliflower
Celery/celery root
Chard
Collards
Cucumber
Eggplant
Garlic
Ginger
Green beans
Horseradish
Jicama
Kale
Leeks
Lettuce, *all leafy greens*
Mushrooms
Onions
Parsnips
Peppers, *all varieties*
Radicchio
Radishes
Rutabaga
Snow/snap peas
Spaghetti squash
Spinach
Tomato
Turnips
Yellow squash
Zucchini

FRUIT
review the Limit foods for more fruit choices!
Lemon
Lime

NUTS/SEEDS
whole, flour, or butters
Almonds
Brazil nuts
Cocoa/cacao (100%), nibs
Chia seeds
Coconut, *all unsweetened forms are okay—coconut sugar is a NO*
Filberts (hazelnuts)
Flax seeds
Hemp seeds
Macadamias
Pecans
Pistachios
Pumpkin seeds
Sunflower seeds
Sesame seeds, tahini
Walnuts

FATS & OILS
review the guide on page 61
Animal fats
Butter, ghee, clarified butter
Avocados, avocado oil
Coconut oil
Flax oil
Olives, olive oil
Sesame oil

DAIRY
full-fat only!
Cheese, cream cheese, cottage cheese
Milk, whole only
Half & half
Heavy cream
Sour cream
Yogurt/kefir, plain

BEVERAGES
Almond milk, unsweetened/homemade (page 213)
Coconut milk, coconut cream, full-fat
Coffee, espresso
Mineral water
Seltzer, club soda
Teas: herbal, green, black, white, etc., unsweetened
Water

CONDIMENTS/MISC.
Broth, homemade only (recipe on page 212)
Coconut aminos
21DSD Ketchup (recipe on page 214)
no store-bought ketchups are allowed
Extracts:
vanilla, almond, etc., and vanilla bean
Hummus made using cauliflower
Healthy Homemade Mayonnaise (recipe on page 211) *do your best to avoid others*
Mustard, gluten-free varieties
Nutritional/Brewer's yeast (Lewis Labs brand)
Salad dressings, homemade
Spices & herbs:
all are OK; check premixed blends for hidden ingredients
Vinegars:
apple cider, balsamic, distilled, red wine, sherry, white

SUPPLEMENTS
Protein powder, 100% pure with NO other ingredients (e.g., 100% whey, egg white, or hemp)
Fermented cod liver oil, with or without flavor (one exception to the no-sweetener rule!)
Pure vitamin or mineral supplements

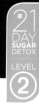

LIMIT FOODS *these are Yes foods with portion size limits*

VEGETABLES & STARCHES
1 cup serving per day is allowed

Acorn squash
Beets
Butternut squash
Green peas
Pumpkin
Winter squash (assorted)

FRUIT
1 piece per day is allowed

Bananas, green-tipped/
  not quite ripe only
Grapefruit
Green/Granny Smith
  apples

BEVERAGES
1 cup total per day is allowed

Coconut juice, coconut
  water: no added sweet-
  eners
Kombucha, home-
  brewed or store-bought
  (see FAQs on pages 46
  and 51, and recom-
  mended brands on
  page 224)

NO FOODS *do not eat these foods for 21 days*

REFINED CARBOHYDRATES
Bagels
Bread
Breadsticks
Brownies
Cake
Candy
Cereal/granola
Chips
Cookies
Couscous
Crackers
Croissants
Cupcakes
Muffins
Oats
Orzo
Pasta
Pastries
Pita
Pizza
Popcorn
Rice cakes
Rolls
Tortillas, tortilla chips

VEGETABLES & STARCHES
Cassava
Corn, polenta, grits
Plantains
Soybeans/edamame
Sweet potatoes/yams
Tapioca, whole & flour
Taro

FRUITS
*review the Yes and Limit foods
lists for the included fruits*
Fresh & dried

GRAINS/LEGUMES
Amaranth
Arrowroot
Barley
Beans: black, fava,
  garbanzo (chickpeas),
  navy, pinto, red
Buckwheat
Flours made from grains
  or beans (chickpeas,
  lentils, etc.)
Kamut
Lentils
Millet
Quinoa
Rice (brown, white, wild)
Rye
Sorghum
Soybeans/edamame
  (including miso, natto,
  tempeh, tofu, and soy
  sauce)
Spelt
Wheat

NUTS/NUT BUTTERS
Cashew
Peanut

SWEETENERS OF ANY KIND
None are allowed! See
page 59 for a complete
list to help you identify
hidden sweeteners.

ANYTHING "DIET," SUGAR-FREE, OR ARTIFICIALLY SWEETENED
This means no gum
either!

SUPPLEMENTS
Anything that includes
  sugar, sweeteners, or
  sugar alcohols (xylitol,
  for example)
Shakeology and other
  similar blends
Supplements that con-
  tain soy, corn, or wheat

BEVERAGES
All alcohol
Coffee "drinks" or shakes,
  pre-sweetened
Juice
Milk: skim, non-fat, 1%,
  2%, soy/rice/oat
Soda (regular & diet)
Sweet-tasting drinks
  (besides herbal teas)
Protein powders that
  have more than one
  ingredient (see Yes food
  supplements)

CONDIMENTS/MISC.
Broth/stock in a box/can
Hummus, made from
  garbanzo beans
Ketchup, store-bought
Mayonnaise, store-bought
Salad dressings, pre-
  made/store-bought
Soy sauce, tamari

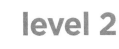
additional notes for those who need more carbohydrates

THESE MODIFICATIONS MAY BE RIGHT FOR YOU IF YOU

- live a very active lifestyle or work at a physically demanding job
- participate in high-intensity physical activity or exercise regularly (for example, interval training, CrossFit-style workouts, endurance athletics, or cardio/aerobic activity at moderate to high intensity for more than 20 minutes at a time; yoga alone doesn't typically require these modifications)
- are pregnant or nursing

With the Energy modifications, you will need to add starchy carbohydrate vegetables to your meal plan that are considered No foods for those who do not fit the modification requirements listed above.

STARCHY CARBOHYDRATE VEGETABLES
amount varies based on your activity level and energy requirements; see page 221 for a list of these foods
Add 30–50 grams of carbohydrates to a *minimum* of one meal per day, especially after exercise. This means 1/2 to 1 cup of mashed sweet potato or plantain, for example. You should also use the one piece of fruit per day included for all Level 2 detoxers to reach this carbohydrate goal.

If you train very hard (at high intensity, or more than once a day), you may need to make this modification for *each instance* of exercise—meaning more than one meal or snack will include up to this amount of dense carbohydrates.

You may adjust what time of day you include your extra carbs. For example, if sweet potato is listed at lunch but you generally feel better including your additional carbs at dinner, you can absolutely do that. In general, adding more carbs later in the day or after activity tends to replenish your fuel better. *This is a highly variable element in your meal planning, and tracking your own energy levels is the best way to decide when to time your extra carbs.*

RECOMMENDED CARBS PER DAY
Moderately active: 75–150 grams
Highly active: 100–200+ grams
Pregnant/nursing: 100+ grams
These are estimates. If you find that you need more carbs to maintain activity, adjust to your needs.

If you are pregnant or nursing one or more children, add these carbohydrate sources as you see fit. Do not limit them assuming it will lead to better results. The goal of this program is a healthy body and a healthy baby, and limiting these foods further is absolutely not necessary! If you find that your milk supply is low or you feel more fatigued than usual, increase your intake of more carbohydrate-dense foods as outlined here.

additional notes for those who eat
seafood, eggs, and dairy, but not meat

THESE MODIFICATIONS MAY BE RIGHT FOR YOU IF YOU
· follow a pescetarian diet

With the Pescetarian modifications, your portion of whole grains or legumes will increase. You will also need to add starchy carbohydrate vegetables to your meal plan that are considered No foods for those who do not fit the modification requirements listed above.

STARCHY CARBOHYDRATE VEGETABLES
you may include up to 2 cups per day; see page 221 for a list of these foods

FULL-FAT DAIRY *no specific portion limits*
You may want to add some high-quality dairy to meals for additional protein and fat. Choose local, grass-fed, and non-homogenized varieties whenever possible. Organic is recommended if you are unable to find grass-fed dairy.

EXTRA FATS
add extra fat portions to meals and snacks
For example:
· add a whole avocado to a meal instead of a half
· add 1/4 cup nuts and/or dressing to a salad instead of 2 tablespoons
· make good use of full-fat dairy products for fat and protein if you tolerate dairy well (tolerating dairy means that you don't experience symptoms such as gas, bloating, digestive distress, acne, eczema, or congestion when you eat it)

SEAFOOD
make seafood your protein source for at least one meal per day, ideally two

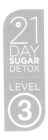

level 3

notes for level 3 that explain its differences from the other levels

While completing The 21-Day Sugar Detox at Level 3, you may choose to follow this meal plan to the letter, follow parts of it to suit your needs or tastes, or simply follow your Yes/No Foods List on page 86-87 along with these general notes.

This level is the most limited in terms of food choices. That said, Level 3 is not recommended simply because you may want to do the "hardest" or "strictest" level of the program. You should have landed here because your answers to the quiz on page 63 determined that this is the right plan for you.

What's different about Level 3 that sets it apart from Levels 1 & 2?
Level 3 excludes all grains and all dairy. This is often referred to as a Paleo type of diet. If you've read my book *Practical Paleo*, then you're familiar with this approach to nutrition. What The 21DSD does that's different from a standard Paleo approach is to remove excess natural sugars and sweet-tasting foods in order to change your habits around sweets and other foods that you rely on habitually.

BALANCEDBITES.COM/21DSD
Printable shopping lists are available online.

level 3

DAY	BREAKFAST	LUNCH	DINNER	SNACK
1 ● ● ▲ ■	buffalo chicken egg muffins (100), steamed spinach, avocado	salmon salad with capers & tomato (154), leafy greens salad or wraps	mini mexi-meatloaves (118), creamy herb mashed cauliflower, *use cilantro* (178)	simple beef jerky (184) + choice of nut mix (192)
2 ● ● ■ ▲	*leftover* buffalo chicken egg muffins, steamed spinach, avocado	*leftover* mini mexi-meatloaves, basic cilantro cauli-rice (172)	broiled salmon with caper & olive tapenade (146), mixed greens salad	*leftover* simple beef jerky + *leftover* nut mix
3 ◆ ▲ ●	green apple breakfast sausage (94), raw carrot sticks, raw almonds	*leftover* broiled salmon, simple spinach & garlic soup (162) or mixed greens with vinaigrette (218)	mustard-glazed chicken thighs (114), golden beets with crispy herbs (180) or green vegetable*	hard-boiled egg + baked kale chips (190)
4 ◆ ● ◆	*leftover* green apple breakfast sausage, raw carrot sticks, raw almonds or walnuts	*leftover* mustard-glazed chicken thighs, *leftover* golden beets with crispy herbs or green vegetable*	asian-style meatballs (138), fresh cabbage & bok choy slaw (171), no-miso soup (164)	21DSD-friendly fruit + nut butter
5 ◆ ◆ ■	bacon & root veggie hash (95), 2 eggs any style or 3oz protein of choice	*leftover* asian-style meatballs, *leftover* cabbage & bok choy slaw	shepherd's pie (134), green salad with dressing of choice (216-218)	grain-free banola (200)
6 ◆ ■ ▲	*leftover* bacon & root veggie hash, 2 eggs any style or 3oz protein of choice	*leftover* shepherd's pie, green salad with dressing of choice (216-218)	shrimp pad thai (148)	*leftover* grain-free banola
7 ▲ ● ▲ ◆	*leftover* shrimp pad thai	perfectly grilled chicken breast (106), broccoli & bacon salad with creamy balsamic dressing (169)	seafood & chorizo paella (142)	simple beef jerky (184) + choice of nut mix (192)

KEY
- ● Eggs
- ● Poultry
- ◆ Pork
- ■ Lamb
- ■ Beef/Bison
- ▲ Seafood

NOTES
*   choose any green vegetable from your Yes foods list on page 86
**   add a starchy vegetable if you are following modifications to do so
Bold italicized items are optional—you can add them or leave them out.
Icons denote the main protein source in meals for your planning purposes. Snacks are optional.

DAY	BREAKFAST	LUNCH	DINNER	SNACK
8 ●●■	tomato-basil quiche with bacon & spinach (104)	*leftover* perfectly grilled chicken breast, lemon & garlic noodles with olives (176)	ginger-garlic beef & broccoli (130), basic cilantro cauli-rice (172)	*leftover* simple beef jerky + *leftover* nut mix
9 ●■♦	*leftover* tomato-basil quiche with bacon & spinach	*leftover* ginger-garlic beef & broccoli, *leftover* basic cilantro cauli-rice	double pork tenderloin (140), green apple & fennel salad (168)	21DSD-friendly fruit + nut butter
10 ●♦▲	lemon chicken with capers & chives (109), raw carrot sticks or steamed vegetables*	*leftover* double pork tenderloin, green salad with dressing of choice (216-218)	lemon sole with almonds & thyme (145), roasted cauliflower soup (160)	21DSD-friendly fruit + nut butter
11 ●▲■	*leftover* lemon chicken with capers & chives, raw carrot sticks or steamed vegetables*	tuna salad wraps (152), *leftover* roasted cauliflower soup or green vegetable*	greek-style meatballs & salad (129), greek tomato & cucumber salad (175)	grain-free banola (200)
12 ♦■●	green apple breakfast sausage (94), raw carrot sticks or other vegetables*	*leftover* greek-style meatballs & salad	hot & sweet ginger-garlic chicken (116), cucumber cold noodle salad (170)	*leftover* grain-free banola
13 ♦●■	*leftover* breakfast sausage, raw carrot sticks, raw almonds or walnuts	*leftover* hot & sweet ginger-garlic chicken, green vegetable*	spaghetti squash bolognese (122), green salad	simple beef jerky (184) + choice of nut mix (192)
14 ●■♦	veggie pancakes (97), 3oz protein of choice	*leftover* spaghetti squash bolognese, green salad	cinnamon grilled pork chops (141), crumb-topped brussels sprouts (181)	*leftover* beef jerky + *leftover* nut mix

KEY
- ● Eggs
- ● Poultry
- ♦ Pork
- ■ Lamb
- ■ Beef/Bison
- ▲ Seafood

NOTES

* choose any green vegetable from your Yes foods list on page 86

** add a starchy vegetable if you are following modifications that direct you to do so

Bold italicized items are optional—you can add them or leave them out.

Icons denote the main protein source in meals for your planning purposes. Snacks are optional.

level 3

DAY	BREAKFAST	LUNCH	DINNER	SNACK
15 ● ◆ ▲	carrot pumpkin spice muffins (103), 2 eggs any style or 3oz protein of choice	*leftover* cinnamon grilled pork chops, *leftover* crumb-topped brussels sprouts	buffalo shrimp lettuce cups (156), basic 4 guacamole (185), jicama fresh "fries" (174)	21DSD-friendly fruit + nut butter
16 ● ● ■ ◆	*leftover* carrot pumpkin spice muffins, 2 eggs any style or 3oz protein of choice	smoky chicken tortilla-less soup (158), *leftover* basic 4 guacamole	stovetop lamb & chorizo chili (136), cocoa-chili roasted cauliflower (179)	21DSD-friendly fruit + nut butter
17 ▲ ■ ◆ ●	rosemary salmon with cabbage (96)	*leftover* stovetop lamb & chorizo chili, *leftover* cocoa-chili roasted cauliflower	chicken with artichokes & olives (110), lemon & garlic noodles with olives (176)	grain-free banola (200)
18 ● ■	smoothie of choice (92-93) with 2 eggs any style or 3oz protein of choice	*leftover* chicken with artichokes & olives, *leftover* lemon & garlic noodles with olives	meatza two-ways (126), pesto spaghetti squash (177)	*leftover* grain-free banola
19 ■ ●	smoothie of choice (92-93) with 2 eggs any style or 3oz protein of choice	[make ahead] italian-style stuffed bell peppers (124)	chicken with tri-color peppers (108), basic cilantro cauli-rice (172)	simple beef jerky (184) + choice of nut mix (192)
20 ● ▲	savory herb drop biscuits (188), 3oz protein of choice, green vegetable*	[make ahead] rainbow collard wraps with herb almond "cheese" spread (150)	spicy sesame-lime salmon (144), cucumber cold noodle salad (170)	*leftover* simple beef jerky + *leftover* nut mix
21 ● ● ■	tomato-basil quiche with bacon & spinach (104)	perfectly grilled chicken breast (106), lemon & garlic noodles with olives (176)	jalapeño bacon burgers (120) with veggie pancakes (97)	21DSD-friendly fruit + nut butter

KEY
● Eggs
● Poultry
◆ Pork
■ Lamb
■ Beef/Bison
▲ Seafood

NOTES

* choose any green vegetable from your Yes foods list on page 86

** add a starchy vegetable if you are following modifications that direct you to do so

Bold italicized items are optional are optional—you can add them or leave them out.

Icons denote the main protein source in meals for your planning purposes. Snacks are optional.

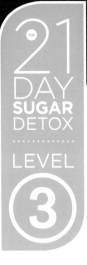

THE
21
DAY
SUGAR
DETOX
....

LEVEL
③

YES FOODS *eat plenty of these foods for 21 days*

MEAT, FISH, & EGGS
including but not limited to:
ALL meats, including deli and
  cured meats like bacon, pancetta, prosciutto, etc. (see
  page 224 for the best brands
  & ingredients to avoid)
ALL seafood
Eggs

VEGETABLES
Artichokes/sunchokes
Asparagus
Broccoli
Brussels sprouts
Cabbage
Carrots
Cauliflower
Celery/celery root
Chard
Collards
Cucumber
Eggplant
Garlic
Ginger
Green beans
Horseradish
Jicama
Kale
Leeks
Lettuce, *all leafy greens*
Mushrooms
Onions
Parsnips
Peppers, *all varieties*
Radicchio
Radishes
Rutabaga
Snow/snap peas
Spaghetti squash
Spinach
Tomato
Turnips
Yellow squash
Zucchini

FRUIT
*review the Limit foods for more
fruit choices!*
Lemon
Lime

NUTS/SEEDS
whole, flour, or butters
Almonds
Brazil nuts
Cocoa/cacao (100%), nibs
Chia seeds
Coconut, *all unsweetened
  forms are okay—coconut
  sugar is a NO*
Filberts (hazelnuts)
Flax seeds
Hemp seeds
Macadamias
Pecans
Pistachios
Pumpkin seeds
Sunflower seeds
Sesame seeds, tahini
Walnuts

FATS & OILS
review the guide on page 61
Animal fats
Butter, ghee, clarified
  butter
Avocados, avocado oil
Coconut oil
Flax oil
Olives, olive oil
Sesame oil

BEVERAGES
Almond milk, unsweetened/
  homemade (page 213)
Coconut milk, coconut
  cream, full-fat
Coffee, espresso
Mineral water
Seltzer, club soda
Teas: herbal, green, black,
  white, etc., unsweetened
Water

CONDIMENTS/MISC.
Broth, homemade only
  (recipe on page 212)
Coconut aminos
21DSD Ketchup (recipe on
  page 214)
  *no store-bought ketchups
  are allowed*
Extracts:
  vanilla, almond, etc., and
  vanilla bean
Hummus made using
  cauliflower
Healthy Homemade Mayon-
  naise (recipe on page 211)
  *do your best to avoid
  others*
Mustard, gluten-free
  varieties
Nutritional/Brewer's yeast
  (Lewis Labs brand)
Salad dressings,
  homemade
Spices & herbs:
  all are OK; check pre-
  mixed blends for hidden
  ingredients
Vinegars:
  apple cider, balsamic,
  distilled, red wine, sherry,
  white

SUPPLEMENTS
Protein powder, 100% pure
  with NO other ingredients
  (i.e. 100% egg white or
  hemp)
Fermented cod liver oil,
  with or without flavor
  (one exception to the no-
  sweetener rule!)
Pure vitamin or mineral
  supplements

**DON'T SEE THE
FOOD YOU WANT TO
EAT ON THE LIST?**
Review "Is it a Yes food?"
on page 65.

MODIFICATIONS
If you are following the
Energy or Autoimmune
track, see the meal plan
modifications on pages
88-89 for additional
notes.

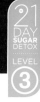

LIMIT FOODS *these are Yes foods with portion size limits*

VEGETABLES & STARCHES
1 cup serving per day is allowed

Acorn squash
Beets
Butternut squash
Green peas
Pumpkin
Winter squash (assorted)

FRUIT
1 piece per day is allowed

Bananas, green-tipped/
  not quite ripe only
Grapefruit
Green/Granny Smith
  apples

BEVERAGES
1 cup total per day is allowed

Coconut juice, coconut
  water:
  no added sweeteners
Kombucha, home-
  brewed or store-bought
  (see FAQs on pages 46
  and 51, and recom-
  mended brands on
  page 224)

NO FOODS *do not eat these foods for 21 days*

REFINED CARBOHYDRATES
Bagels
Bread
Breadsticks
Brownies
Cake
Candy
Cereal/granola
Chips
Cookies
Couscous
Crackers
Croissants
Cupcakes
Muffins
Oats
Orzo
Pasta
Pastries
Pita
Pizza
Popcorn
Rice cakes
Rolls
Tortillas, tortilla chips

VEGETABLES & STARCHES
Cassava
Corn, polenta, grits
Plantains
Soybeans/edamame
Sweet potatoes/yams
Tapioca, whole & flour
Taro

FRUITS
*review the Yes and Limit foods
lists for the included fruits*
Fresh & dried

GRAINS/LEGUMES
Amaranth
Arrowroot
Barley
Beans: black, fava,
  garbanzo (chickpeas),
  navy, pinto, red
Buckwheat
Flours made from grains
  or beans (chickpeas,
  lentils, etc.)
Kamut
Lentils
Millet
Quinoa
Rice (brown, white, wild)
Rye
Sorghum
Soybeans/edamame
  (including miso, natto,
  tempeh, tofu, and soy
  sauce)
Spelt
Wheat

NUTS/NUT BUTTERS
Cashew
Peanut

DAIRY
Cheese, cream cheese,
  cottage cheese
Milk
Half & half
Heavy cream
Sour cream
Yogurt/kefir

SWEETENERS OF ANY KIND
None are allowed! See
page 59 for a complete
list to help you identify
hidden sweeteners.

ANYTHING "DIET," SUGAR-FREE, OR ARTIFICIALLY SWEETENED
This means no gum
either!

SUPPLEMENTS
Anything that includes
  sugar, sweeteners, or
  sugar alcohols (xylitol,
  for example)
Shakeology and other
  similar blends
Supplements that con-
  tain soy, corn, or wheat

BEVERAGES
All alcohol
Coffee "drinks" or shakes,
  pre-sweetened
Juice
Milk, soy/rice/oat
Soda (regular & diet)
Sweet-tasting drinks
  (besides herbal teas)
Protein powders that
  have more than one
  ingredient (see Yes food
  supplements)

CONDIMENTS/MISC.
Broth/stock in a box/can
Hummus, made from
  garbanzo beans
Ketchup, store-bought
Mayonnaise, store-bought
Salad dressings, pre-
  made/store-bought
Soy sauce, tamari

additional notes for those who need more carbohydrates

THESE MODIFICATIONS MAY BE RIGHT FOR YOU IF YOU

· live a very active lifestyle or work at a physically demanding job
· participate in high-intensity physical activity or exercise regularly (for example, interval training, CrossFit-style workouts, endurance athletics, or cardio/aerobic activity at moderate to high intensity for more than 20 minutes at a time; yoga alone doesn't typically require these modifications)
· are pregnant or nursing

With the Energy modifications, you will need to add starchy carbohydrate vegetables to your meal plan that are considered No foods for those who do not fit the modification requirements listed above.

STARCHY CARBOHYDRATE VEGETABLES
amount varies based on your activity level and energy requirements; see page 221 for a list of these foods
Add 30–50 grams of carbohydrates to a *minimum* of one meal per day, especially after exercise. This means 1/2 to 1 cup of mashed sweet potato or plantain, for example. You should also use the one piece of fruit per day included for all Level 3 detoxers to reach this carbohydrate goal.

If you train very hard (at high intensity, or more than once a day), you may need to make this modification for *each instance* of exercise—meaning more than one meal or snack will include up to this amount of dense carbohydrates.

You may adjust what time of day you include your extra carbs. For example, if sweet potato is listed at lunch but you generally feel better including your additional carbs at dinner, you can absolutely do that. In general, adding more carbs later in the day or after activity tends to replenish your fuel better. *This is a highly variable element in your meal planning, and tracking your own energy levels is the best way to decide when to time your extra carbs.*

RECOMMENDED CARBS PER DAY
Moderately active: 75–150 grams
Highly active: 100–200+ grams
Pregnant/nursing: 100+ grams
These are estimates. If you find that you need more carbs to maintain activity, adjust to your needs.

If you are pregnant or nursing one or more children, add these carbohydrate sources as you see fit. Do not limit them assuming it will lead to better results. The goal of this program is a healthy body and a healthy baby, and limiting these foods further is absolutely not necessary! If you find that your milk supply is low or you feel more fatigued than usual, increase your intake of carbohydrate-dense foods as outlined here.

MODIFICATIONS **autoimmune** level 3

additional notes for those who have
autoimmune health conditions

THESE MODIFICATIONS MAY BE RIGHT FOR YOU IF YOU

• have been diagnosed with an autoimmune condition or suspect you may have one

With the Autoimmune modifications, you will be eliminating several foods from your meal plan that are considered Yes foods for those who do not fit the modification requirements listed above. These foods are common allergens and are often generally irritating to digestion. By improving digestive function, immune function can also be improved. If you have an autoimmune condition and have never eliminated these foods, I highly recommend doing so for the 21 days of this program to see how you feel without them, then reintroduce them and track any changes.

EGGS
omit from your meals and snacks
See page 222 for egg-free breakfast ideas!

NUTS & SEEDS
omit from your meals and snacks
This includes whole nuts, nut butters, seeds, and seed butters. Nuts are highlighted in recipes where they are included, and omissions or substitutions are noted if the recipe can bear the change.

NIGHTSHADE VEGETABLES & SPICES
omit from your meals and snacks
This includes tomatoes, potatoes, peppers (including spices such as paprika, chili powder, and cayenne pepper), and eggplant. Nightshades are highlighted in recipes where they are included, and omissions or substitutions are noted if the recipe can bear the change.

easy **recipes**

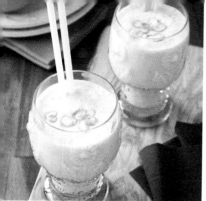
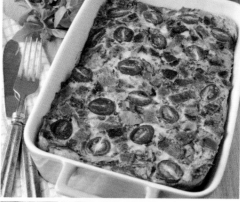
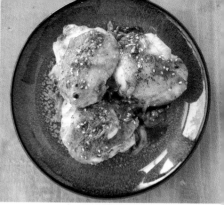
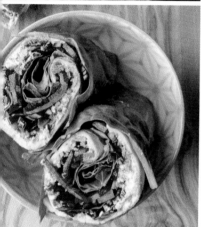
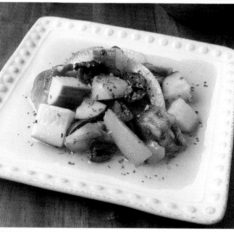
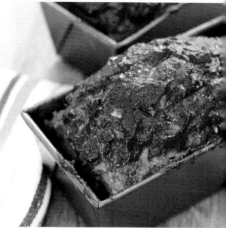
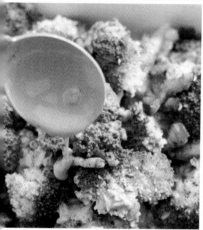
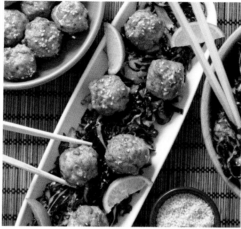
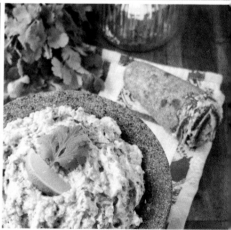
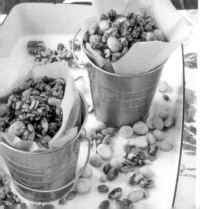
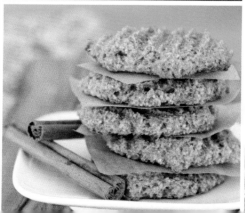
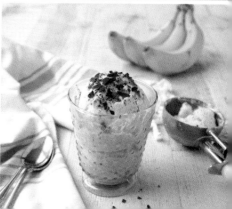

almond milk smoothies

PREP TIME **5 MINS** • SERVINGS **1-2**

NUTS

EGGS

NIGHTSHADES

FODMAPS

SEAFOOD

COCO-MONKEY SMOOTHIE

1/4 avocado

1 cup almond milk (page 213)

1 green-tipped banana, frozen

3 tablespoons unsweetened cocoa powder*

2 tablespoons almond meal, store-bought* or homemade (page 213)

pinch of ground cinnamon

small handful of ice (optional)

ALMOND AVO-NANA SMOOTHIE

1/4 avocado

1 cup almond milk (page 213)

1 green-tipped banana, frozen

1/4 teaspoon ground cinnamon

2 tablespoons almond meal, store-bought* or homemade (page 213)

small handful of ice (optional)

INGREDIENT TIP
*Check out page 224 for a list of recommended brands. ●

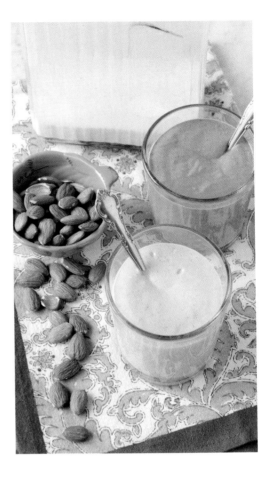

Purée all the ingredients in a blender until smooth.

coconut milk smoothies

PREP TIME **5 MINS** • SERVINGS **1-2**

ZESTY CREAMSICLE SMOOTHIE

1 cup full-fat coconut milk*
1/2 cup water
1 green-tipped banana, frozen
seeds scraped from 1/4 vanilla bean pod
zest of 1 orange
small handful of ice (optional)

LIME IN THE COCONUT SMOOTHIE

1 cup full-fat coconut milk*
1/2 cup water
1 green-tipped banana, frozen
1 teaspoon lime zest
juice of 1/2 lime
small handful of ice (optional)

INGREDIENT TIP
*Check out page 224 for a list of recommended brands. ●

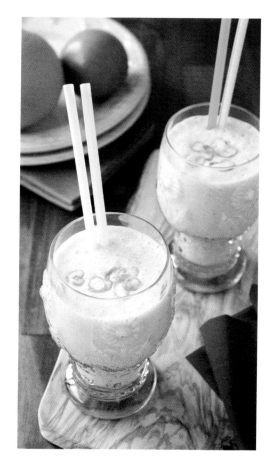

NUTS

EGGS

NIGHTSHADES

FODMAPS

SEAFOOD

Purée all the ingredients in a blender until smooth.

green apple breakfast sausage

PREP TIME **10 MINS** • COOK TIME **10-12 MINS** • SERVINGS **4**

NUTS

EGGS

NIGHTSHADES

FODMAPS

SEAFOOD

1 pound ground pork, beef, chicken, or turkey

1/2 green apple, peeled and diced

2 tablespoons Italian Sausage Spice Blend (page 208)

In a mixing bowl, combine the ground meat, apple, and Italian Sausage Spice Blend and mix with your hands until the spices and apples are evenly incorporated. Form the mixture into 8 evenly sized patties.

Heat a large skillet over medium heat. When hot, place the patties in the pan and cook for 5 to 6 minutes per side or until cooked through and browned.

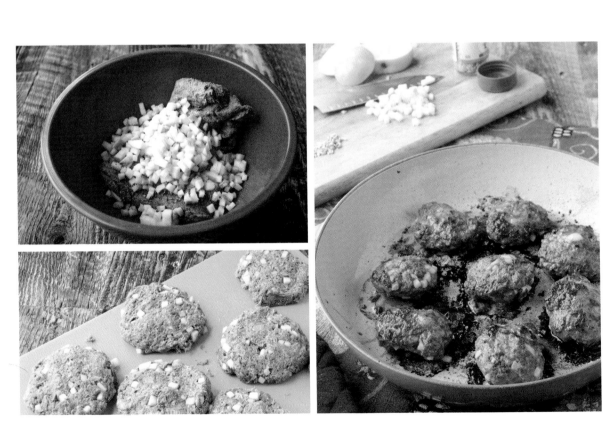

bacon & root veggie hash

PREP TIME **15 MINS** • COOK TIME **20 MINS** • SERVINGS **4**

4 slices bacon

1 shallot, minced

4 cups grated parsnips
(approximately 8 medium)

1/4 cup grated carrots

1 tablespoon Italian Sausage
Spice Blend (page 208)

FODMAP FREE?
Omit the shallot. ●

Slice the bacon crosswise into 1/4-inch strips. In a large skillet over medium heat, cook the bacon until the fat is rendered and the meat is cooked, approximately 10 minutes. Remove the bacon from the pan and drain on paper towels, leaving the fat in the pan.

Add the shallot to the pan and cook for 2 minutes or until it becomes translucent. Add the parsnips, carrots, and Italian Sausage Spice Blend to the pan and continue to cook until the vegetables are soft and cooked through, 5 to 8 minutes.

Add the bacon back to the pan and toss to combine and heat through.

Serve with eggs (any style), your favorite breakfast sausage links, or Green Apple Breakfast Sausage (page 94).

NUTS

EGGS

NIGHTSHADES

FODMAPS

SEAFOOD

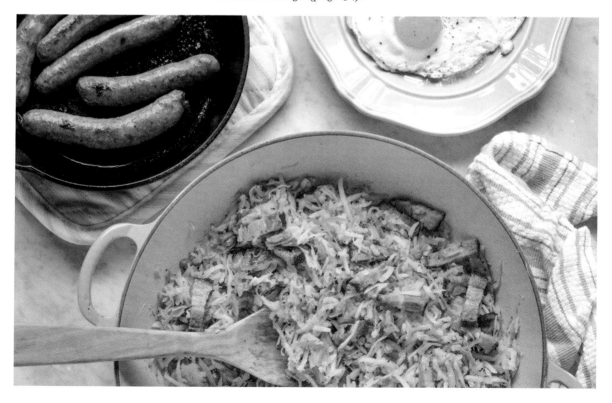

NUTS

EGGS

NIGHTSHADES

FODMAPS

SEAFOOD

rosemary salmon with cabbage

PREP TIME **10 MINS** • COOK TIME **12 MINS** • SERVINGS **4**

FOR THE SALMON
1 teaspoon dried rosemary

1 teaspoon sea salt

1/2 teaspoon black pepper

1 pound wild salmon fillets

2 tablespoons ghee or coconut oil, melted

1 lemon, thinly sliced into rounds

FOR THE CABBAGE
1 head green cabbage

2 tablespoons coconut oil

1 teaspoon apple cider vinegar

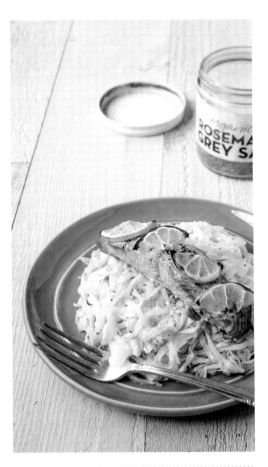

Place the oven rack in the top position and preheat the broiler to low.

In a small mixing bowl, combine the rosemary, salt, and pepper.

Place the salmon in an oven-safe dish and brush evenly with a thin layer of the ghee or coconut oil, then sprinkle half of the spice blend evenly over the salmon. Top the salmon with the lemon slices.

Broil for 8 to 12 minutes, depending on the thickness of the salmon. (The rule of thumb is 10 minutes per inch.)

While the salmon broils, halve the cabbage through its core, then quarter it and remove the core. Slice the cabbage crosswise as thinly as possible. In a large skillet over medium heat, melt the coconut oil, then add the cabbage, vinegar, and the remaining spice blend. Sauté until soft, 8 to 10 minutes.

To serve, create a bed of cabbage on each plate and top with the salmon.

veggie pancakes

PREP TIME **10 MINS** • COOK TIME **20 MINS** • SERVINGS **6-8**

- 4 cups grated zucchini (4 small or 2 large) or carrots
- 3 eggs, beaten
- 1/2 teaspoon granulated garlic
- 1/4 cup coconut flour
- 1/2 teaspoon sea salt
- 1/2 teaspoon black pepper
- 1/4 cup ghee, coconut oil, or bacon fat

NUTS

EGGS

NIGHTSHADES

FODMAPS

SEAFOOD

CHEF NOTE
Check out page 121 to see these pancakes made with carrots and used as a burger bun. ●

Place the zucchini or carrots in the center of a large piece of cheesecloth or a mesh fabric bag, then bundle up the fabric around the vegetable, twist, and squeeze out any excess water.

In a large mixing bowl, combine the eggs, granulated garlic, salt, and pepper; then sift in the coconut flour and mix well. Stir in the vegetables.

In a large skillet, heat the ghee, coconut oil, or bacon fat over medium-low heat. Using a 1/4-cup measure, place the vegetable mixture into the hot skillet and cook for 3 to 4 minutes. Gently flip the pancakes and cook for 3 to 4 minutes on the other side. Repeat with the remaining vegetable mixture.

These pancakes are more delicate when warm but become a bit firmer when they cool to room temperature or are chilled—making them ideal faux burger buns (see page 121).

pumpkin pancakes
with vanilla bean coconut butter

PREP TIME **5 MINS** • COOK TIME **30 MINS** • SERVINGS **4**

NUTS

EGGS

NIGHTSHADES

FODMAPS

SEAFOOD

FOR THE PANCAKES

6 eggs

3/4 cup canned pumpkin

1 1/2 teaspoons pure vanilla extract

1 1/2 teaspoons pumpkin pie spice

1 1/2 teaspoons cinnamon

3 tablespoons coconut flour

1/4 teaspoon baking soda

pinch of sea salt

3 tablespoons ghee or coconut oil, divided

FOR THE VANILLA BEAN COCONUT BUTTER

3 tablespoons coconut butter,* softened

3/4 teaspoon pure vanilla extract

seeds from 1/2 vanilla bean pod

INGREDIENT TIP
*Check out page 224 for a list of recommended brands.

KITCHEN TIP
If you are using freshly cooked or boxed pumpkin purée in this recipe, strain the excess water by placing it in cheesecloth over a bowl and refrigerate overnight before using it. ●

In a large mixing bowl, whisk the eggs, pumpkin, and vanilla. Sift the pumpkin pie spice, cinnamon, coconut flour, baking soda, and salt into the wet ingredients. Alternative option: Pulse all the ingredients in a food processor until well mixed.

Grease a skillet with 1 teaspoon of the ghee or coconut oil and spoon the batter into the skillet to make pancakes of your desired size. Allow the pancakes to cook for about 3 minutes, and when a few bubbles appear, flip the pancakes and cook for another 3 minutes. Repeat with the remaining batter, greasing the pan each time.

Make the Vanilla Bean Coconut Butter: Combine the coconut butter, vanilla, and vanilla bean seeds in a small mixing bowl. Mix well to combine, then use to top pancakes.

Alternate topping ideas: almond butter, sliced green bananas, chopped walnuts or pecans.

Serve with bacon or sausage.

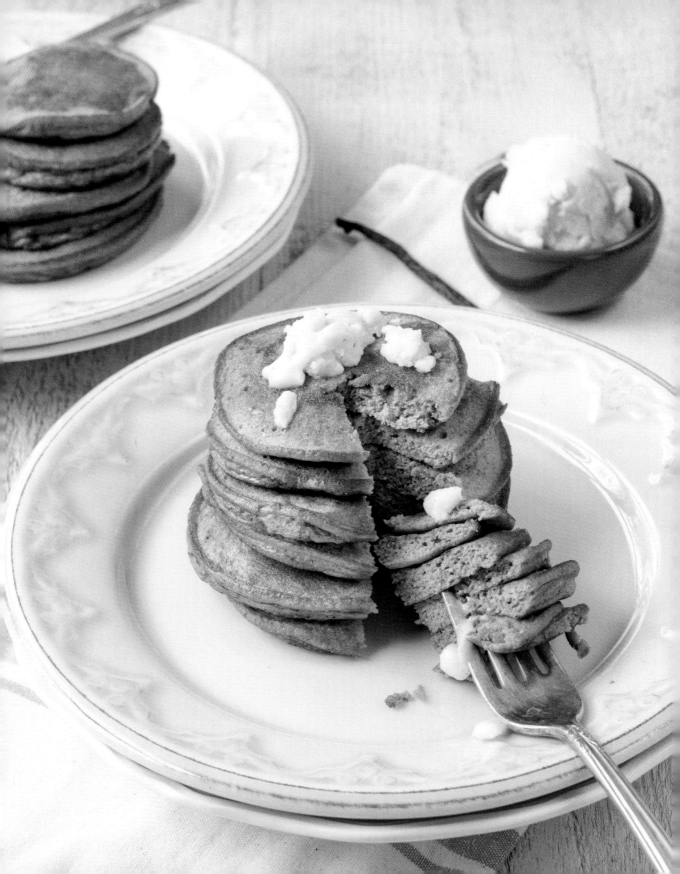

buffalo chicken egg muffins

PREP TIME **10 MINS** • COOK TIME **50 MINS** • SERVINGS **6** • YIELD **12 MUFFINS**

NUTS

EGGS

NIGHTSHADES

FODMAPS

SEAFOOD

1 1/2 pounds boneless, skinless chicken thighs or breasts

1 teaspoon granulated garlic

1/2 teaspoon sea salt

1/2 teaspoon black pepper

1/2 cup Tessemae's Wing Sauce, divided, or 1/4 cup other clean ingredient hot sauce* and 1/4 cup melted unsalted butter or coconut oil

12 large eggs

1/4 cup sliced green onions (scallions)

sea salt and black pepper to taste

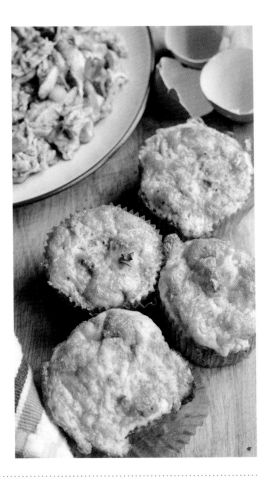

INGREDIENT TIP

*If you can't find Tessemae's Wing Sauce, my favorite organic gluten-free hot sauce is from Arizona Gunslinger—chipotle habañero flavor—available online and in many specialty grocery stores and co-ops. Check out page 224 for more 21DSD-friendly brands of sauces and condiments.

EQUIPMENT TIP

For the parchment paper muffin cup liners, see Recommended Products & Brands on page 224. ●

Preheat the oven to 425°F. Prepare 12 cups of a muffin tin with parchment paper muffin cup liners.

Arrange the chicken on a baking sheet and season with the granulated garlic, salt, and pepper. Bake for 25 minutes or until cooked through.

Working in a large bowl, shred the chicken by pulling the meat apart with 2 forks. Pour 1/4 cup of the wing sauce over the chicken and toss to combine.

In a mixing bowl, whisk the eggs, the remaining 1/4 cup wing sauce, green onions, salt, and pepper.

Pour the egg mixture into the muffin cups, filling them approximately halfway. Gently spoon about 1/4 cup of the shredded chicken into each muffin cup. Serve any extra chicken alongside the cooked muffins.

Bake for 40 minutes or until the muffins rise and become golden brown around the edges.

broccoli & herb egg muffins

PREP TIME **10 MINS** • COOK TIME **30 MINS** • SERVINGS **4** • YIELD **8 MUFFINS**

1 cup broccoli, chopped into 2-inch florets

8 eggs

1 cup fresh cilantro (or other herb)

2 teaspoons onion powder

1/2 teaspoon sea salt

1/2 teaspoon black pepper, or more to taste

1 teaspoon dulse flakes (optional)

NUTS
EGGS
NIGHTSHADES
FODMAPS
SEAFOOD

EQUIPMENT TIP
For the parchment paper muffin cup liners, see Recommended Products & Brands on page 224. ⬤

Preheat oven to 350°F. Prepare 8 cups of a muffin tin with parchment paper muffin cup liners.

Place the broccoli in a small saucepan or pot filled with 1 inch of water over high heat. Steam the broccoli for 2 to 5 minutes or until bright green and fork-tender. Set aside to cool a bit.

In a blender, combine the eggs, cilantro, onion powder, salt, pepper, and dulse flakes, if using.

Add the broccoli florets and pulse to combine.

Pour the mixture evenly into the prepared muffin cups.

Bake for 30 minutes or until the muffins rise and become golden brown around the edges.

apple streusel egg muffins

PREP TIME **10 MINS** • COOK TIME **40 MINS** • SERVINGS **3** • YIELD **6 MUFFINS**

NUTS

EGGS

NIGHTSHADES

FODMAPS

SEAFOOD

1 tablespoon coconut oil, butter, or ghee

1 1/2 cups peeled & chopped green apple

1 1/2 teaspoons cinnamon, divided

3 tablespoons warm water

6 eggs

2 tablespoons full-fat coconut milk*

1/2 teaspoon pure vanilla extract

1/4 teaspoon apple cider vinegar

1 tablespoon coconut flour

1/4 teaspoon baking soda

pinch of sea salt

INGREDIENT TIP
*Check out page 224 for a list of recommended brands.

EQUIPMENT TIP
For the parchment paper muffin cup liners, see Recommended Products & Brands on page 224. ●

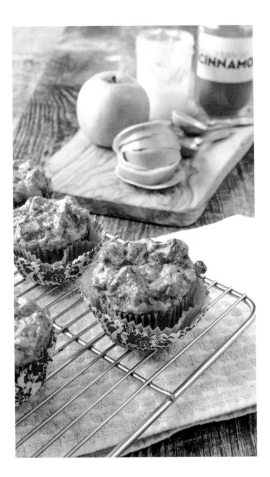

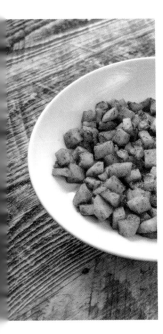

Preheat the oven to 350°F.

In a medium skillet, melt the coconut oil, butter, or ghee over medium heat. Then sauté the apples, 1 teaspoon of the cinnamon, and water until the apples are the consistency of chunky applesauce or apple pie filling. Set aside to cool completely.

In a medium-sized mixing bowl, whisk together the eggs, coconut milk, vanilla, and vinegar. Sift in the coconut flour, the remaining 1/2 teaspoon cinnamon, baking soda, and salt and whisk until well combined. Stir in the cooled apples, reserving 1/4 cup for garnish.

Prepare 6 cups of a muffin tin with parchment paper muffin cup liners. Pour the egg and apple mixture evenly into the lined muffin cups. Gently spoon about 1 teaspoon of the remaining apple mixture onto the top of each muffin.

Bake for 40 minutes or until the muffins rise and become golden brown around the edges.

carrot pumpkin spice muffins

PREP TIME **15 MINS** • COOK TIME **35-40 MINS** • SERVINGS **12** • YIELD **12 MUFFINS**

6 eggs, beaten

1/4 cup canned pumpkin

1/2 cup unsalted butter, ghee, or coconut oil, melted

1 teaspoon pure vanilla extract

1 green-tipped banana, mashed

1/2 cup coconut flour

pinch of sea salt

1/4 teaspoon baking soda

1 tablespoon pumpkin pie spice

3 cups grated carrots (approximately 4 large)

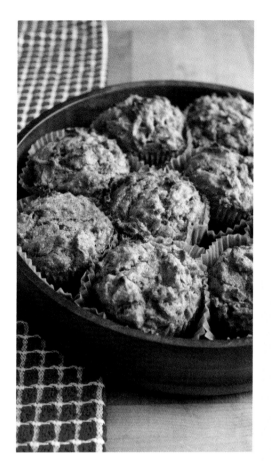

NUTS

EGGS

NIGHTSHADES

FODMAPS

SEAFOOD

EQUIPMENT TIP
For the parchment paper muffin cup liners, see Recommended Products & Brands on page 224.

KITCHEN TIP
If you are using freshly cooked or boxed pumpkin purée, strain the excess water by placing it in a cheesecloth over a bowl and refrigerate overnight before using it.

AFTER THE 21DSD
Add 1/4 cup of raisins or cranberries when you stir in the carrots—remember, no dried fruit if you are making these for The 21DSD! ●

Preheat the oven to 350°F.

In a large mixing bowl, whisk together the eggs; pumpkin; butter, ghee, or coconut oil; vanilla; and banana. Sift in the coconut flour, salt, baking soda, and pumpkin pie spice and stir until well combined. Gently fold in the carrots.

Prepare 12 cups of a muffin tin with parchment paper muffin cup liners. Scoop 1/4 cup of the batter into each muffin cup.

Bake for 35 to 40 minutes or until the muffins are golden brown and a toothpick inserted into the center comes out clean.

tomato-basil quiche
with bacon & spinach

PREP TIME **15 MINS** • COOK TIME **40-50 MINS** • SERVINGS **4**

NUTS

EGGS

NIGHTSHADES

FODMAPS

SEAFOOD

8 slices bacon

8 eggs

2 cloves garlic, minced or grated

2 tablespoons chopped fresh chives

1/4 cup chopped fresh basil leaves

1/2 teaspoon sea salt

1 teaspoon black pepper

2 cups chopped spinach

1 to 2 tablespoons bacon fat (reserved from cooking bacon)

12 cherry tomatoes, halved

Preheat the oven to 375°F.

Slice the bacon crosswise into 1/4-inch strips. In a skillet over medium heat, cook the bacon until the fat is rendered and the meat is cooked, approximately 8 to 10 minutes. Remove the bacon from the pan and drain on paper towels; reserve the fat.

In a large mixing bowl, whisk the eggs, garlic, chives, basil, salt, and pepper until well combined. Stir in the spinach.

Grease a 9 by 11-inch baking dish with the reserved bacon fat, then pour the egg mixture into the pan. Top with the bacon pieces and cherry tomato halves.

Bake for 30 to 35 minutes or until the quiche puffs up and becomes golden brown on the edges.

NIGHTSHADE FREE?
Omit the cherry tomatoes. ●

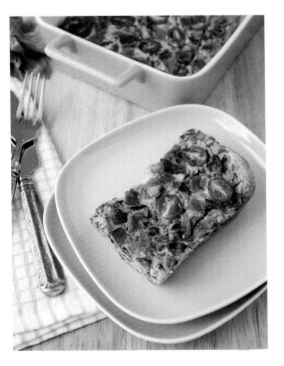

THE 21-DAY SUGAR DETOX • DIANE SANFILIPPO

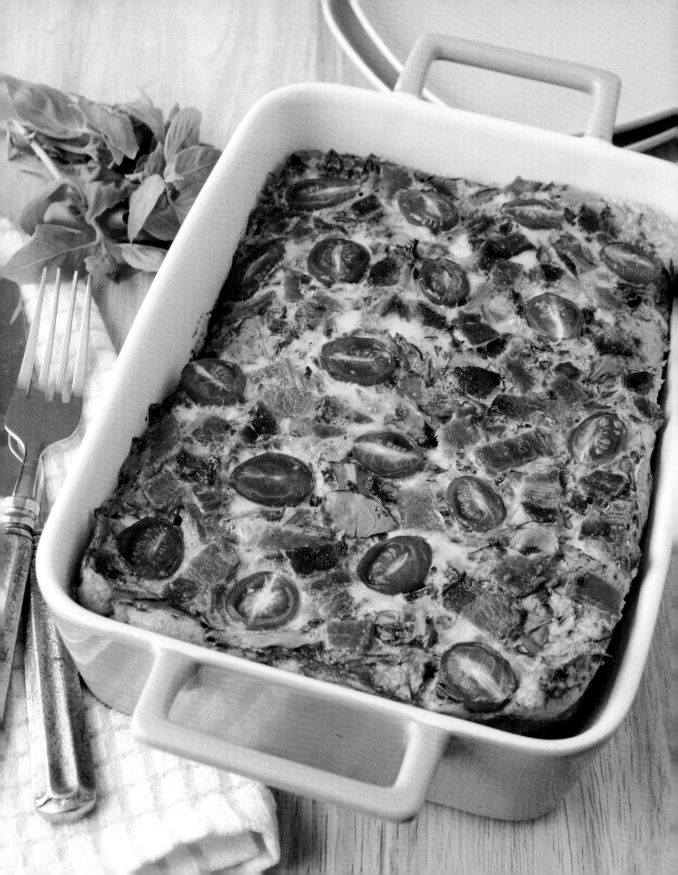

perfectly grilled chicken breast

PREP TIME **10-15 MINS** • COOK TIME **10 MINS** • SERVINGS **4**

NUTS

EGGS

NIGHTSHADES

FODMAPS

SEAFOOD

1 pound boneless, skinless chicken breast

juice of 1 lemon, or 2 tablespoons balsamic vinegar

1 teaspoon dried oregano, rosemary, or other herb

1/2 teaspoon sea salt

1/2 teaspoon black pepper

2 tablespoons coconut oil or ghee

2 tablespoons extra-virgin olive oil

Preheat a grill pan or grill to medium heat.

Place a chicken breast on a cutting board with the thickest side facing you. Set your non-cutting hand on top and, while pressing down slightly on the chicken with your palm (keeping your fingers out straight), begin cutting down the length of the side of the breast, keeping your knife parallel to the cutting board. Carefully slide the knife through the center so that the thickness is cut in half. Continue to slice almost completely through the chicken breast, leaving it connected in the center so that it flattens out to a "butterfly" or heart shape—see the top piece of chicken pictured at right. The chicken should now be 1/4- to 1/2-inch thick at most. Repeat with the remaining chicken breasts.

In a large bowl, combine the lemon juice or vinegar with the oregano, salt, and pepper. Add the chicken and turn to evenly coat; allow to marinate for at least 5 minutes, but not more than an hour.

Brush the hot grill or grill pan with the coconut oil or ghee, then cook the chicken for 4 to 5 minutes per side, depending on the thickness of the chicken. When you notice that the chicken has turned white up around the sides and toward the middle, it's time to flip it.

When you take the chicken off the grill, brush it liberally with the extra-virgin olive oil. Allow to sit for at least 5 minutes before slicing to eat.

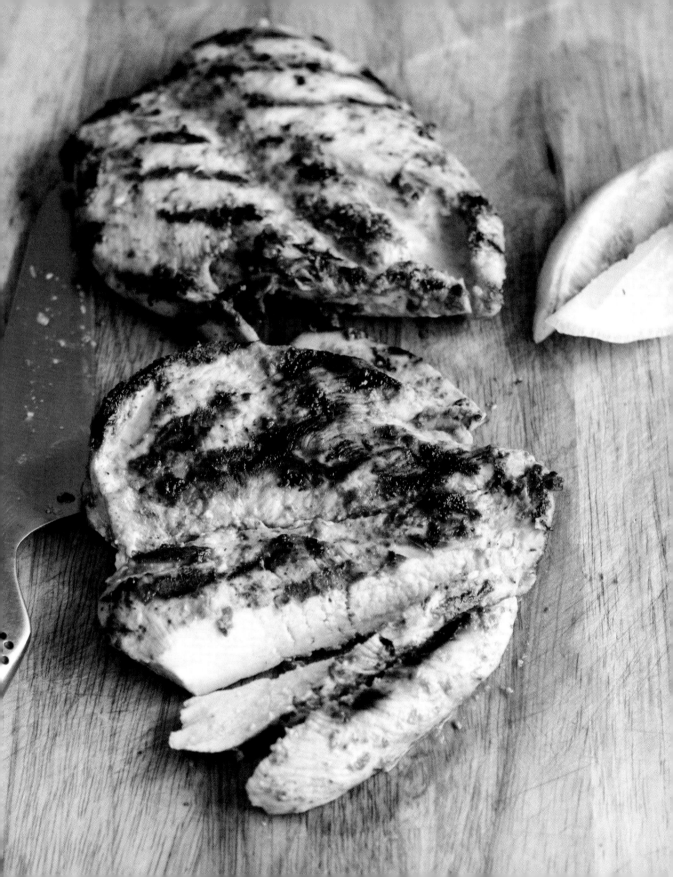

chicken with tri-color peppers

PREP TIME **10 MINS** • COOK TIME **40-50 MINS** • SERVINGS **4**

NUTS

EGGS

NIGHTSHADES

FODMAPS

SEAFOOD

1 red bell pepper

1 poblano pepper*

1 banana pepper*

2 teaspoons duck fat, coconut oil, or unsalted butter

1 teaspoon sea salt, divided

1 teaspoon black pepper, divided

1/2 cup Bone Broth, chicken (page 212)

4 chicken leg quarters

1/2 teaspoon onion powder

1/2 teaspoon granulated garlic

INGREDIENT TIP

*If you can't find banana and poblano peppers, just use any three different-colored peppers you can find that are within a heat/spiciness range that you enjoy. ●

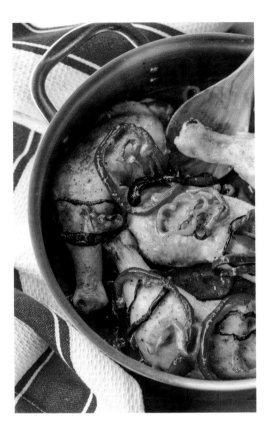

Preheat the oven to 400°F.

Slice each of the peppers into rings that are approximately 1/8- to 1/4-inch thick, removing the white core and seeds.

In a large, oven-safe sauté pan, melt the duck fat, coconut oil, or butter over medium heat, then add the sliced peppers and season with 1/2 teaspoon of the salt and 1/2 teaspoon of the pepper. Allow the peppers to cook until they soften and the edges become slightly browned and just barely begin to stick to the pan. Pour in the Bone Broth to deglaze the pan and stir gently to release any brown bits from the bottom of the pan.

Season the chicken leg quarters with the onion powder, granulated garlic, the remaining 1/2 teaspoon salt, and the remaining 1/2 teaspoon pepper. Slide the peppers to the sides of the sauté pan. Place the chicken in the pan, and arrange the pepper slices on top of the chicken.

Place the pan in the oven and bake for 30 minutes or until the chicken reaches 165°F when a thermometer is inserted into the thickest part of the meat.

lemon chicken with capers & chives

PREP TIME **10 MINS** • COOK TIME **45-60 MINS** • SERVINGS **4-6**

1 whole (4- to 6-pound) chicken (or bone-in, skin-on parts if you prefer)

2 tablespoons ghee, unsalted butter, duck fat, or coconut oil, melted

1/2 cup capers, drained

1/4 cup chopped fresh chives

1 lemon, zested and sliced into rounds

sea salt and black pepper to taste

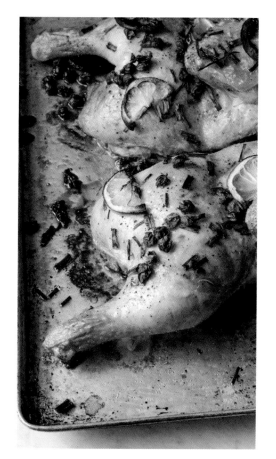

NUTS

EGGS

NIGHTSHADES

FODMAPS

SEAFOOD

Preheat the oven to 425°F.

Split the chicken in half using a large chef's knife, then lay it flat on a rimmed baking sheet, skin side up.

Brush the skin generously with the ghee, then sprinkle on the capers, chives, and lemon zest. Season liberally with salt and pepper, then place the lemon slices on the chicken.

Roast for 45 to 60 minutes or until the internal temperature of the chicken reaches 165°F. The cooking time will vary based on the size of the chicken or the bone-in parts you select.

chicken with artichokes & olives

PREP TIME **15 MINS** • COOK TIME **35-40 MINS** • SERVINGS **4**

NUTS

EGGS

NIGHTSHADES

FODMAPS

SEAFOOD

- 4 tablespoons ghee or unsalted butter, divided
- 4 cups frozen or canned artichoke hearts, defrosted/drained
- 1 cup pitted olives (mix of green and kalamata)
- 1/2 cup olive brine (from olives above)
- 8 bone-in, skin-on chicken thighs
- 2 teaspoons ground turmeric
- 2 teaspoons granulated garlic
- 1 teaspoon ground cumin
- 1 teaspoon ground coriander
- 1/4 teaspoon sea salt, or more to taste
- 1/4 teaspoon black pepper, or more to taste
- 1 lemon
- 1 teaspoon red chili flakes (optional; omit for nightshade free)

Preheat the oven to 425°F.

Grease a large oven-safe casserole dish or clay pot with 2 tablespoons of the ghee or butter, then place the artichoke hearts, olives, and olive brine in the pan. Place the chicken thighs on top.

In small mixing bowl, combine the turmeric, granulated garlic, cumin, coriander, salt, and pepper. Sprinkle enough of the spice blend over the chicken to coat the skin well, then distribute the rest over the artichoke hearts and olives. Top each chicken thigh with a small dollop of ghee or butter—about 3/4 teaspoon.

Cut half of the lemon into thin rounds and place them around the pan; squeeze the other half over the entire pan. Sprinkle with the red chili flakes, if using.

Bake, covered, for 20 minutes, then remove the lid and bake for another 15 to 20 minutes or until the internal temperature of the chicken reaches 165°F.

CHEF NOTE

If bone-in, skin-on thighs aren't your favorite cut, you can make this recipe with chicken breasts, leg quarters, or drumsticks.

ON THE SIDE

This recipe pairs well with a green salad or can be served over Basic Cilantro Cauli-Rice (page 172). ●

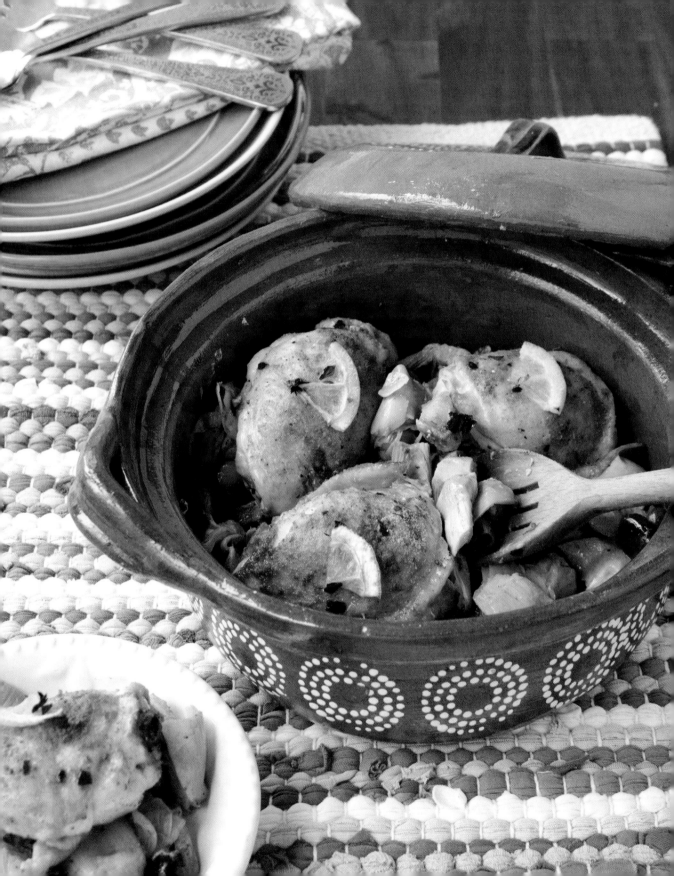

parsnip & bacon stuffed chicken roll-ups

PREP TIME **20 MINS** • COOK TIME **60 MINS** • SERVINGS **4**

NUTS

EGGS

NIGHTSHADES

FODMAPS

SEAFOOD

4 slices bacon

4 cups roughly chopped parsnips

1 teaspoon bacon fat (reserved from cooking bacon) or coconut oil

1 small shallot, minced

2 green onions (scallions), chopped

2 pounds boneless, skinless chicken thighs (approximately 8 pieces)

sea salt and black pepper to taste

FODMAP FREE?
Omit the green onions. ●

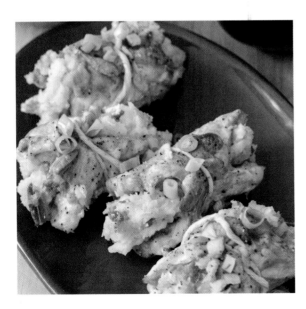

Preheat the oven to 350°F.

Set the bacon on a rack over a rimmed baking sheet and bake for 20 to 30 minutes or until cooked through. Set the cooked bacon aside and reserve the bacon fat. When the bacon is cool, chop it into 1/4-inch pieces.

While the bacon bakes, steam the parsnips in a basket over 1 inch of water until fork-tender, 8 to 10 minutes. Purée the parsnips in a food processor or mash them by hand with a fork or a potato masher. Place the mashed parsnips in a mixing bowl and set aside.

Increase the oven temperature to 400°F.

In a small skillet, heat the bacon fat over medium heat. Sauté the shallot until it is translucent and the edges are just beginning to brown.

Fold the shallots, green onions, and chopped bacon into the mashed parsnips. Season with salt and pepper to taste. Set the filling mixture aside.

Place the chicken thighs on a cutting board and pound them out with a mallet—striking the meat in a down-and-outward motion to create a larger area—until the meat is less than 1/4-inch thick.

Season both sides of the chicken liberally with salt and pepper, then set a 6-inch piece of cooking twine under each flattened piece. Spoon 2 to 4 tablespoons of the mashed parsnips into the center of each piece of chicken. Fold the chicken up and over the filling and secure with the twine. Transfer the roll-ups to a deep oven-safe dish or cast-iron skillet and place in the oven. Roast for 30 minutes or until the internal temperature of the stuffing reaches 165° F.

Serve with any extra parsnip purée on the side along with a green salad.

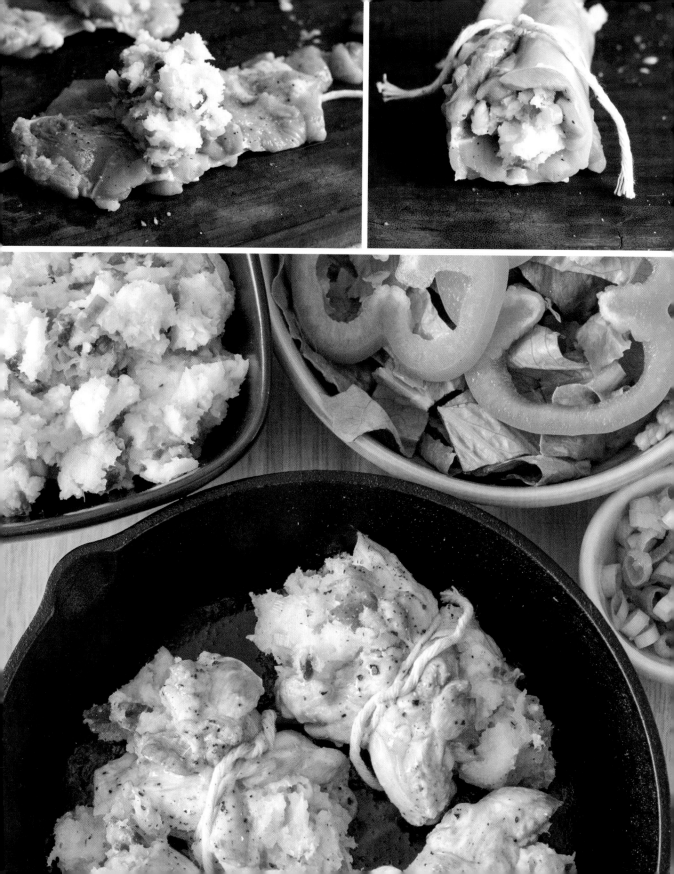

mustard-glazed chicken thighs

PREP TIME **25 MINS** • COOK TIME **45 MINS** • SERVINGS **4**

NUTS

EGGS

NIGHTSHADES

FODMAPS

SEAFOOD

1/4 cup melted unsalted butter or coconut oil

2 tablespoons gluten-free mustard*

1/2 teaspoon dried sage

1/2 teaspoon sea salt

black pepper to taste

8 bone-in, skin-on chicken thighs

Preheat the oven to 425°F.

In a small mixing bowl, combine the melted butter or coconut oil, mustard, sage, salt, and pepper. Place the chicken thighs on a rimmed baking sheet or in a large baking dish, and brush the mustard glaze evenly over each one.

Bake for 45 minutes or until a thermometer reads 165°F when inserted into the center of one of the chicken thighs.

INGREDIENT TIP
*Check out page 224 for a list of recommended brands.

KITCHEN TIP
Use bone-in, skin-on chicken breasts if you don't have chicken thighs. Serve with Creamy Herb Mashed Cauliflower (page 178) and a green salad. These are fantastic reheated in the oven or toaster oven, and they make a delicious breakfast as well.

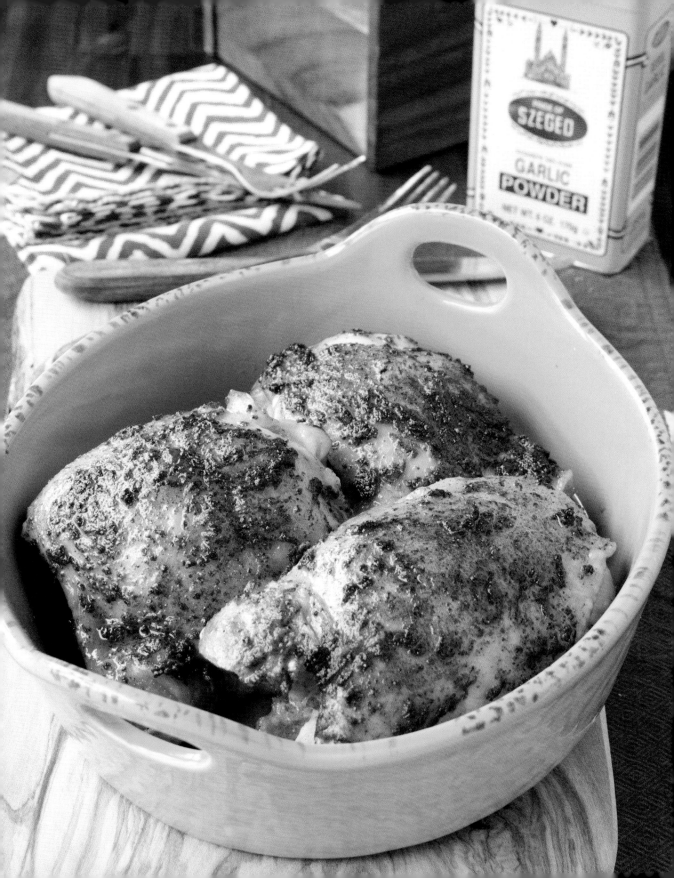

hot & sweet ginger-garlic chicken

PREP TIME **5 MINS** • COOK TIME **30-35 MINS** • SERVINGS **4**

NUTS

EGGS

NIGHTSHADES

FODMAPS

SEAFOOD

- 1 tablespoon ghee or coconut oil
- 8 bone-in, skin-on chicken thighs, or 4 bone-in, skin-on chicken breasts
- sea salt and black pepper to taste
- 1 medium onion, finely sliced
- 2 cloves garlic, minced
- 1 teaspoon ginger powder or minced fresh ginger
- 2 teaspoons white sesame seeds
- 1 teaspoon red chili flakes, or to taste
- 1/3 cup coconut aminos*

INGREDIENT TIP
*Check out page 224 for a list of recommended brands.

NIGHTSHADE FREE?
Leave out the chili flakes. ●

Preheat the oven to 425°F.

In an oven-safe cast-iron or stainless-steel skillet, melt the ghee or coconut oil. Season both sides of the chicken with salt and pepper, and place the pieces skin side down in the pan. Roast for 5 to 6 minutes or until the skin browns and releases easily from the pan.

While the chicken cooks, combine the onion, garlic, ginger, sesame seeds, chili flakes, coconut aminos, and more salt and pepper in a small mixing bowl.

Flip the chicken thighs over so that they are skin side up in the pan. Pour the sauce mixture evenly over the chicken and bake for 30 minutes or until the internal temperature of the chicken reaches 165°F.

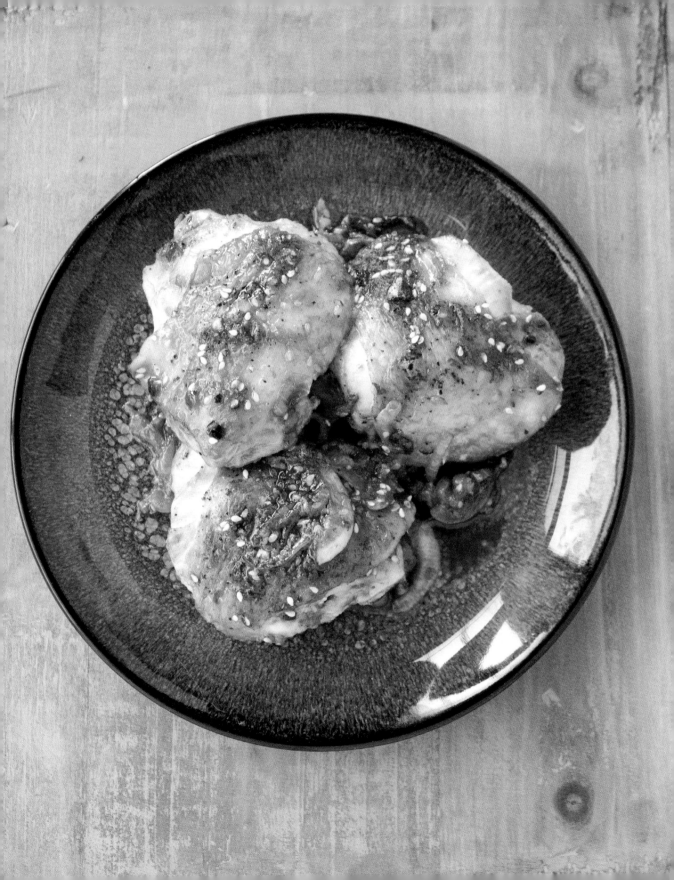

mini mexi-meatloaves

PREP TIME **25 MINS** • COOK TIME **40-50 MINS** • SERVINGS **4-6**

FOR THE SAUCE

7 ounces tomato paste

1/2 cup water

1/4 cup chopped red bell pepper

1 tablespoon chopped fresh cilantro leaves

1/2 teaspoon chili powder

1/4 teaspoon sea salt

black pepper to taste

FOR THE MEATLOAF MIXTURE

1 tablespoon coconut oil, duck fat, or bacon fat

1 small onion, chopped (about 1/2 cup)

2 cloves garlic, minced or grated

1 teaspoon ground cumin

1 teaspoon ground coriander

1 teaspoon chili powder

1/2 teaspoon sea salt

1/4 teaspoon black pepper

2 carrots, grated

1 bell pepper, any color, grated or very finely chopped

1/4 cup chopped fresh cilantro leaves

2 eggs, beaten

2 pounds ground beef

Preheat the oven to 375°F. Line 2 mini loaf pans or 1 regular-sized loaf pan with parchment paper.

Make the sauce: In a small saucepan over medium-low heat, combine the tomato paste, water, bell pepper, cilantro, chili powder, salt, and pepper. Simmer for 5 to 10 minutes, stirring occasionally to prevent burning. If the sauce reduces too far and looks like it may burn, add more water, 2 tablespoons at a time, and whisk to combine. The sauce should be fairly thick, almost like ketchup, not loose like a pasta sauce.

While the sauce is simmering, prepare the meatloaf mixture: In a medium skillet, melt the coconut oil or duck or bacon fat over medium-low heat. Cook the onion until it is translucent and the edges begin to brown, then add the garlic and stir for about a minute.

In a large mixing bowl, combine the cooked onion and garlic, cumin, coriander, chili powder, salt, pepper, carrots, bell pepper, and cilantro; mix well. Add the eggs and ground beef and, using your hands, mix everything together until well combined.

Divide the meatloaf mixture into the 2 prepared mini loaf pans or place it all in the prepared regular-sized loaf pan, filling the pan(s) up to and slightly over the top, as the mixture will shrink a bit in cooking.

Spoon about 1/4 cup of the sauce onto each mini loaf, or 1/2 cup onto the single loaf, spreading it in an even layer to coat the top. Reserve the remaining amount for dipping after the loaves are baked.

Bake, uncovered, for 40 to 50 minutes (60 to 70 minutes for the single, large loaf) or until the internal temperature reaches 160°F.

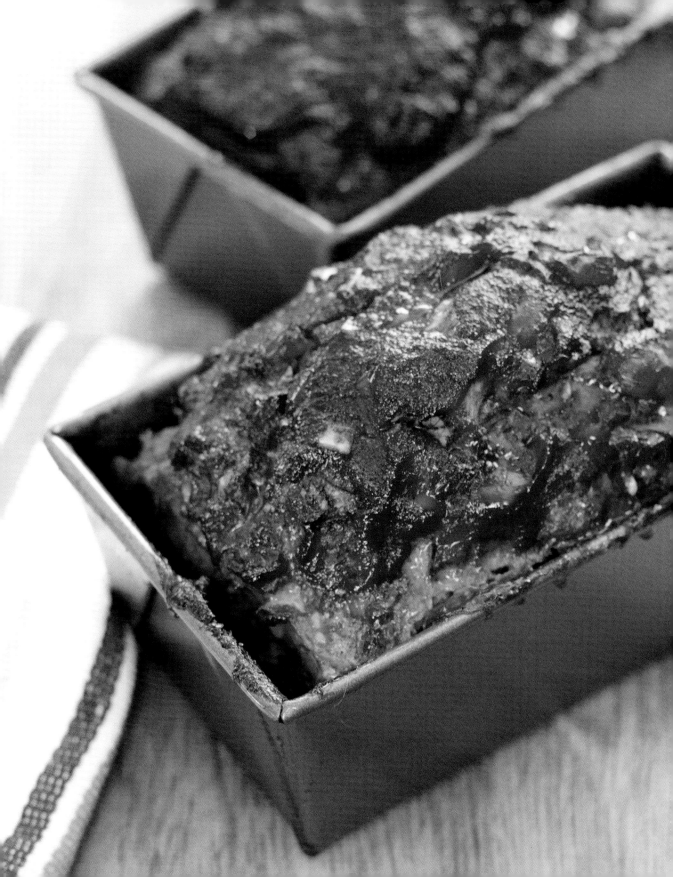

jalapeño bacon burgers

PREP TIME **15 MINS** • COOK TIME **8-12 MINS** • SERVINGS **4**

NUTS

EGGS

NIGHTSHADES

FODMAPS

SEAFOOD

8 slices bacon, divided

1 jalapeño pepper

1 pound ground beef, bison, or turkey

1 tablespoon Smoky Spice Blend (page 208)

Several slices red onion

FOR THE BUNS

1 recipe Veggie Pancakes (page 97) or large lettuce leaves, for use as "buns" (optional)

Preheat a grill or grill pan to medium-high heat.

Cut 6 slices of the bacon into 1/8-inch square pieces. (The remaining 2 slices will be used for the topping.)

Slice the jalapeño in half lengthwise, then remove the seeds and white membrane. If you like a lot of heat, you may leave the white part intact or even use the seeds. Finely chop the jalapeño.

In a mixing bowl, combine the ground meat, bacon pieces, Smoky Spice Blend, and jalapeño. Form into 4 evenly sized patties, then place on the hot grill or grill pan. Cook for 5 to 6 minutes per side, depending on your desired level of doneness.

While the burgers grill, cook the 2 reserved bacon slices in a small skillet over medium heat until browned.

Serve with Veggie Pancakes as "buns" or wrapped in lettuce. Top with the red onion and cooked bacon slices.

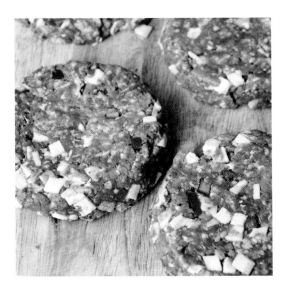

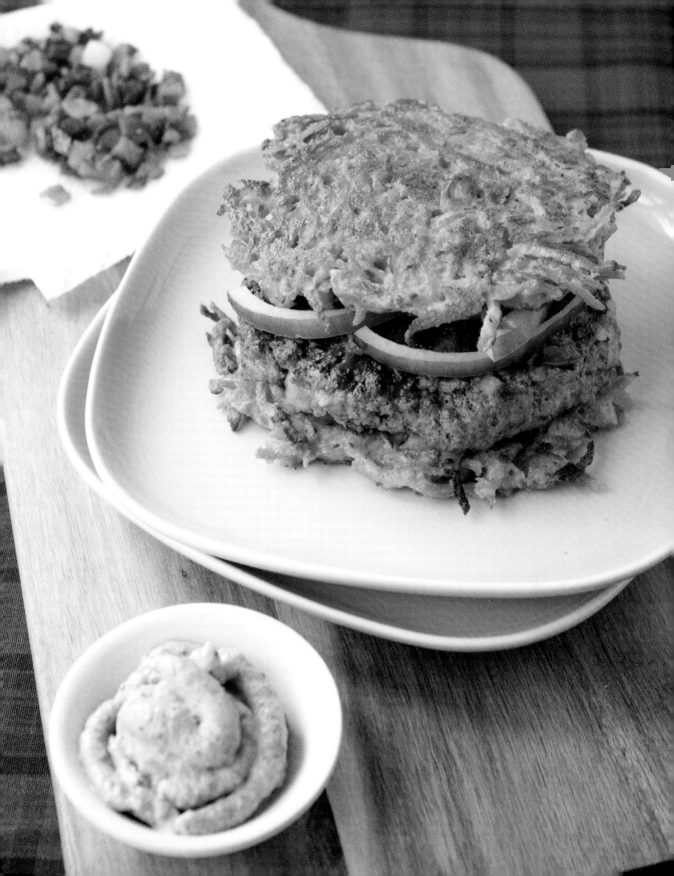

spaghetti squash bolognese

PREP TIME **15 MINS** • COOK TIME **45 MINS** • SERVINGS **4**

1 spaghetti squash (3 to 4 pounds)

sea salt and black pepper to taste

FOR THE SAUCE

2 tablespoons bacon fat or unsalted butter

1 onion, diced

1 carrot, diced

1 celery stalk, finely diced

1 clove garlic, minced or grated

1/2 pound ground veal or beef

1/2 pound ground pork

4 slices bacon, chopped

1/2 cup full-fat coconut milk*

3 ounces tomato paste

sea salt and black pepper to taste

INGREDIENT TIP

*Check out page 224 for a list of recommended brands.

NIGHTSHADE FREE?

Try making this dish with canned pumpkin instead of tomato paste! ●

Preheat the oven to 375°F.

Slice the spaghetti squash in half lengthwise. Scoop the seeds and inner membranes out of the hollows, then sprinkle liberally with salt and pepper. Place both halves facedown on a rimmed baking sheet. Roast for 35 to 45 minutes or until the flesh of the squash becomes translucent and the skin begins to soften and separate from the "noodles" that make up the inside. Allow the squash to cool enough that you can handle it, then scoop out the flesh into a large serving bowl.

While the squash bakes, make the sauce: In a large skillet over medium-high heat, melt the bacon fat or butter. Sauté the onion, carrot, and celery until they become translucent, then add the garlic and cook for an additional minute.

Add the ground veal or beef, ground pork, and bacon and cook until browned and cooked through, approximately 10 to 12 minutes. Add the coconut milk and tomato paste and simmer over medium-low heat for 20 to 30 minutes.

Add the salt and pepper before removing the sauce from the heat.

Serve over the roasted spaghetti squash.

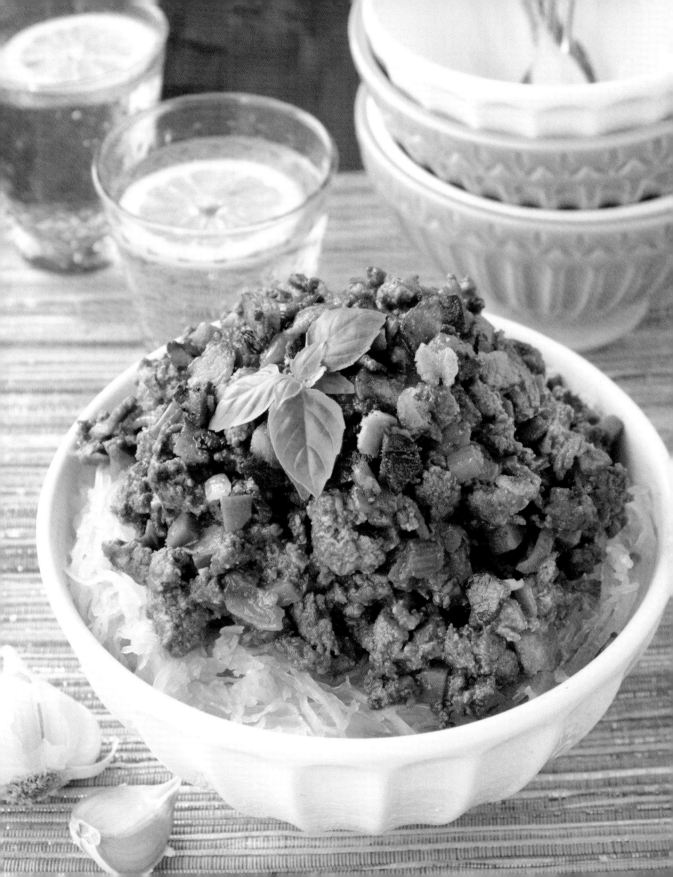

italian-style stuffed bell peppers

PREP TIME **20 MINS** • COOK TIME **25-35 MINS** • SERVINGS **4**

NUTS

EGGS

NIGHTSHADES

FODMAPS

SEAFOOD

2 bell peppers, halved, cored, and seeded

1 tablespoon bacon grease or coconut oil

1/2 large onion, diced

sea salt and black pepper

4 cloves garlic, minced or grated

1/2 cup diced tomatoes, fresh or canned

1 pound ground beef, bison, turkey, or chicken

6 fresh basil leaves, minced, plus extra for garnish

Preheat the oven to 375°F.

Place the bell pepper halves facedown in a roasting dish or an oven-safe skillet and bake for 10 to 15 minutes. (You can skip this step if you want to keep the peppers more firm/raw.)

While the bell peppers are cooking, heat the bacon grease or coconut oil in a large skillet over medium-high heat. Sauté the onion, adding salt and pepper to taste, until it is translucent and slightly browned on the edges. Reduce the heat to medium, add the garlic and tomatoes, and cook for about 2 minutes.

Add the meat and cook until fully done. Taste the mixture, and add more salt or pepper if needed. Mix in the basil.

Remove the peppers from the oven—they should be just a bit softened—and flip them over. Spoon the stuffing mixture into each one. You can go ahead and eat them at this point, or put them back in the oven for 15 to 20 minutes to allow the flavors of the bell pepper and the meat mixture to blend. Garnish with basil leaves and serve.

You can refrigerate or freeze these to reheat later.

COOKING TIP

It's best not to use acidic ingredients (like tomatoes or vinegar) in cast-iron cookware since the acid will interact with the iron. This is a good time to use an enameled cast-iron or stainless-steel skillet or a ceramic roasting dish.

CHANGE IT UP

Add 2 cups chopped baby spinach to the meat.

NIGHTSHADE FREE?

Stuff summer squash or portobello mushrooms instead of peppers, and omit the tomatoes.

FODMAP FREE?

Omit the onions and garlic and stuff the mixture into squash instead of peppers. ●

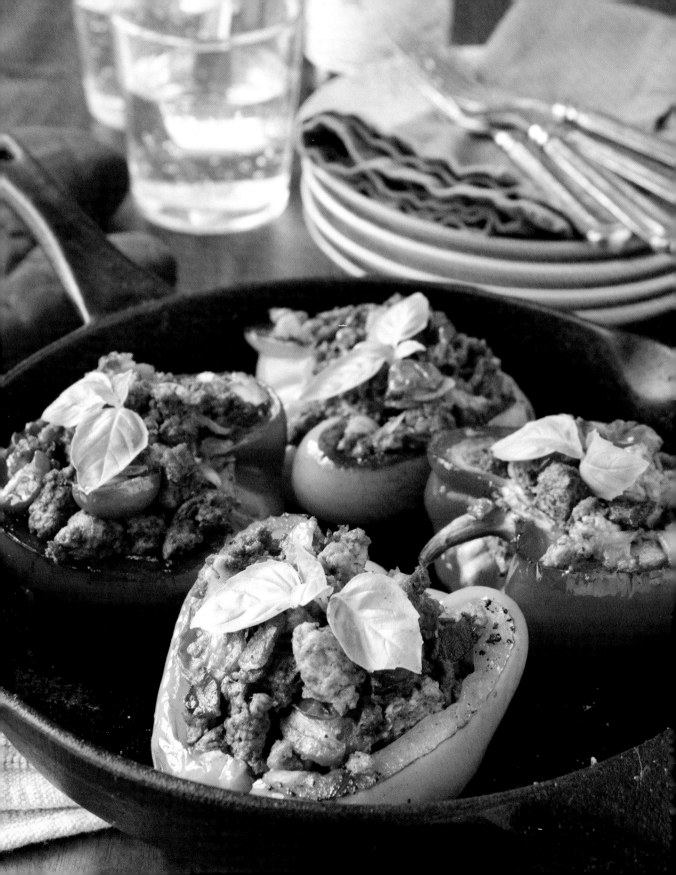

meatza two-ways

PREP TIME **30 MINS** • COOK TIME **40 MINS** • SERVINGS **4-6**

FOR THE CRUSTS

1 pound ground beef

1 pound ground pork

2 eggs, beaten (optional)

2 tablespoons almond meal, store-bought* or homemade (page 213) (optional)

2 teaspoons granulated garlic

2 teaspoons onion powder

2 teaspoons dried oregano

1 teaspoon fennel seeds, crushed (optional)

2 teaspoons sea salt

1 teaspoon black pepper

FOR THE TOPPINGS

(or use any of your favorites!)

1 head garlic, roasted and mashed (see Kitchen Tip)

1 large tomato, thinly sliced

1/4 cup sliced artichoke hearts

1/4 cup pitted and sliced kalamata olives

2 tablespoons coconut oil or ghee

1 small zucchini, sliced

1 small eggplant, sliced

1 bell pepper, sliced

1 tablespoon dried oregano, for garnish

For Levels 1 and 2, add cheese if you like

INGREDIENT TIP

*Check out page 224 for a list of recommended brands.

KITCHEN TIP

To make roasted garlic, slice the top and bottom off of a whole garlic bulb, then top with 2 tablespoons of cooking fat, wrap securely in aluminum foil, and bake at 350°F for approximately 40 minutes.

Preheat the oven to 350°F.

If you plan to use roasted garlic as a topping, pop it in the oven now, as it takes 40 minutes to roast (see Kitchen Tip).

Make the crusts: In a mixing bowl, combine the beef, pork, eggs, almond meal (if using), granulated garlic, onion powder, oregano, fennel, salt, and pepper; mix until well incorporated.

Divide the meat mixture into four 8-ounce portions and form into crusts approximately 6 inches across and 1/4-inch thick. Bake on a rimmed sheet for 15 to 20 minutes or until cooked through. Remove the crusts from the oven and set aside.

While the crusts are baking, prepare the toppings. If you choose to grill your vegetable toppings (zucchini, eggplant, and bell pepper), brush a grill or grill pan with coconut oil and preheat it to medium-high heat. Cook the vegetables for approximately 3 minutes per side.

Increase the oven temperature to 425°F.

Top the meatza crusts with the toppings of your choice, then place back in the oven for 5 to 10 minutes or until the toppings soften just a bit.

TOPPINGS PICTURED:
Sliced tomato, grilled eggplant, and grilled bell pepper (TOP).

Roasted garlic, grilled zucchini, sliced artichoke hearts, and sliced kalamata olives (BOTTOM, nightshade free).

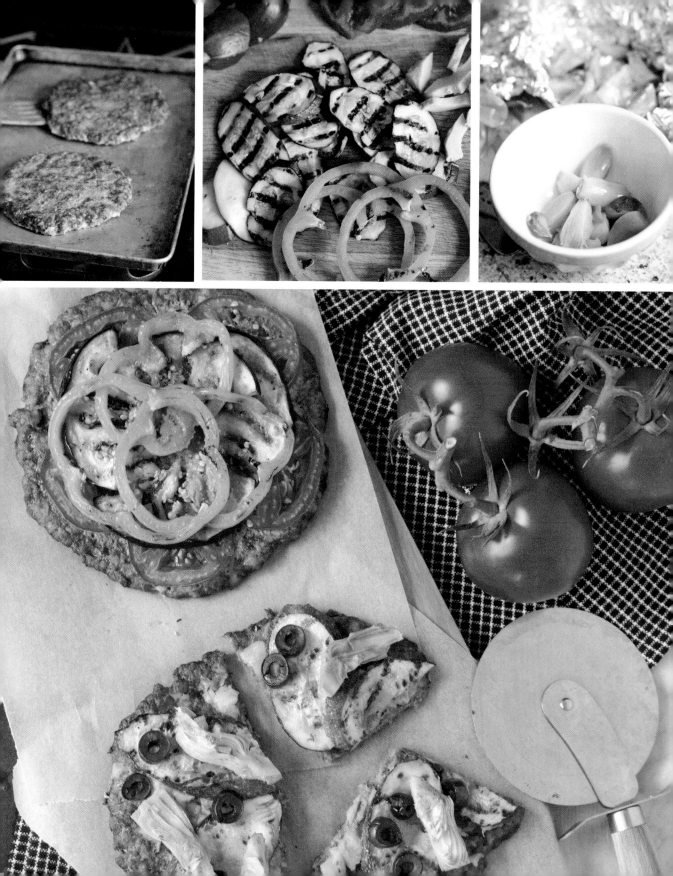

balsamic-braised beef

PREP TIME **5 MINS** • COOK TIME **8 HRS** • SERVINGS **4**

NUTS

EGGS

NIGHTSHADES

FODMAPS

SEAFOOD

- 3 to 4 pounds beef short ribs, or 2 pounds boneless beef such as stew meat or a roast
- 5 to 6 large cloves garlic, peeled or smashed
- 1 medium yellow onion, roughly chopped
- 4 large carrots, peeled and roughly sliced
- 1 (14.5-ounce) can diced tomatoes
- 1/4 cup water
- 1/2 cup balsamic vinegar
- 1/2 teaspoon sea salt, plus more to taste
- 1/2 teaspoon black pepper, plus more to taste

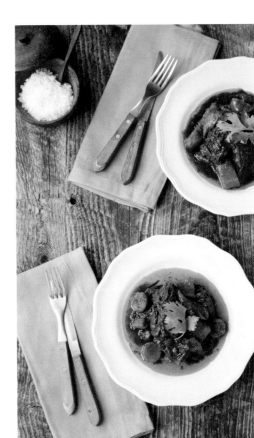

ON THE SIDE
This dish pairs perfectly with Creamy Herb Mashed Cauliflower (page 178). ●

Place all the ingredients in a slow cooker set on low for 8 or more hours until the meat falls apart easily with a fork. Taste and add more salt and pepper if needed.

Alternative directions: If you don't have a slow cooker, preheat the oven to 200°F, place all the ingredients in a large enameled cast-iron Dutch oven, and cook for 6 hours or until the meat falls apart easily with a fork.

greek-style meatballs & salad

PREP TIME **15 MINS** • COOK TIME **25 MINS** • SERVINGS **3-4**

1 pound ground lamb, beef, or turkey

1 large clove garlic, minced or grated

zest of 1 lemon

1/2 teaspoon dried oregano

1/4 teaspoon granulated garlic

1/2 teaspoon sea salt

1/4 teaspoon black pepper

1 lemon, sliced into thin rounds

1 to 2 tablespoons extra-virgin olive oil

FOR THE SALAD

1 head or 2 hearts romaine lettuce, chopped

1 cup frozen or canned artichoke hearts, defrosted/drained

1 large tomato, sliced

1/4 cup pitted and halved kalamata olives

juice of 1 lemon (from zested lemon above)

1/4 cup extra-virgin olive oil

1 teaspoon dried oregano

NUTS

EGGS

NIGHTSHADES

FODMAPS

SEAFOOD

NIGHTSHADE FREE?
Omit the tomatoes.

Preheat the oven to 400°F.

In a mixing bowl, combine the ground meat, garlic, lemon zest, oregano, granulated garlic, salt, and pepper; mix well to thoroughly incorporate the spices and salt into the meat.

Form the meat mixture into 9 to 12 meatballs and place in a baking dish. Place the lemon slices in the pan on top of some of the meatballs.

Bake for 20 to 25 minutes or until the meatballs are cooked all the way through or are just slightly pink in the center.

Drizzle the extra-virgin olive oil over the meatballs upon serving.

Make the salad: Place the lettuce in a large serving bowl and top with the artichoke hearts, tomato slices, and olives. In a small bowl, whisk together the lemon juice, olive oil, and oregano and pour over the salad.

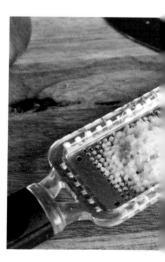

ginger-garlic beef & broccoli

PREP TIME **15 MINS** • COOK TIME **10 MINS** • SERVINGS **3-4**

NUTS

EGGS

NIGHTSHADES

FODMAPS

SEAFOOD

FOR THE MARINADE

1/4 cup coconut aminos*

2 to 3 drops fish sauce*

2 tablespoons minced shallot

2 tablespoons sliced green onion (scallion)

1/2 teaspoon minced fresh ginger

1 teaspoon minced or grated garlic

1/2 teaspoon sea salt

1/2 teaspoon black pepper

1 pound skirt steak

1 large head broccoli, chopped into 1- to 2-inch pieces

1 teaspoon coconut oil or ghee

OPTIONAL GARNISHES

1 tablespoon white sesame seeds

1/4 cup finely sliced red cabbage

1/4 cup sliced green onions (scallions)

INGREDIENT TIP
*Check out page 224 for a list of recommended brands.

ON THE SIDE
This recipe pairs well with Basic Cilantro Cauli-Rice (page 172). ●

In a mixing bowl, whisk together the ingredients for the marinade.

Lay the skirt steak flat on a cutting board and cut with the grain to divide it into sections that are approximately 4 inches long. Then cut against the grain to slice the meat into 1/4-inch wide strips.

Set the meat in a large, flat pan and pour the marinade over the top, turning the meat to coat it. Let it marinate for 10 minutes.

While the steak marinates, set up a pot with 1 inch of water and a steamer basket. Steam the broccoli for 8 to 10 minutes or until bright green and still slightly firm. Transfer to a colander to drain off any excess moisture.

In a large skillet, melt the coconut oil or ghee over medium-high heat. Place the steak and the marinating liquid in the pan and cook for approximately 1 minute per side or until cooked through. When the meat is just about finished, add the broccoli and gently toss to combine and heat through.

Garnish with white sesame seeds, red cabbage, and/or green onions, if using.

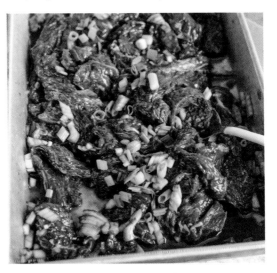

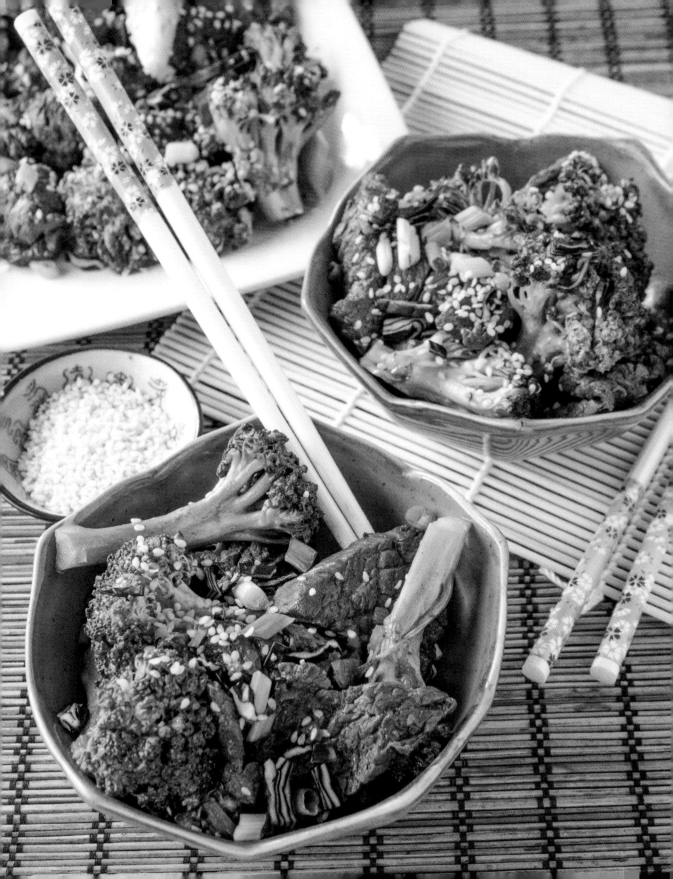

crunchy curried beef lettuce cups

PREP TIME **15 MINS** • COOK TIME **25 MINS** • SERVINGS **3-4**

NUTS

EGGS

NIGHTSHADES

FODMAPS

SEAFOOD

1 tablespoon ghee or coconut oil

1 cup chopped jicama

1/2 cup chopped bell pepper

2 tablespoons minced shallot

sea salt and black pepper to taste

2 tablespoons curry powder

1/4 teaspoon ginger powder, or 1/2 teaspoon minced fresh ginger

1/2 teaspoon onion powder

1 teaspoon ground cinnamon

1 clove garlic, minced or grated

1/4 cup full-fat coconut milk*

1 pound ground beef

juice of 1 lime

1/4 cup chopped fresh cilantro leaves

1 head butter or Bibb lettuce, separated into leaves

1 lime, cut into wedges, for garnish

OPTIONAL GARNISHES

1/4 cup finely sliced red cabbage

1/4 cup sliced green onions (scallions)

fresh basil leaves

In a large skillet, melt the ghee or coconut oil over medium-high heat. Place the jicama, bell pepper, and shallot in the pan and season with salt and pepper. When the vegetables begin to soften—approximately 5 to 10 minutes— add the curry powder, ginger, onion powder, cinnamon, and garlic. Stir to combine and coat the vegetables with the spices.

Continue to sauté for 5 minutes, then stir in the coconut milk. Add the ground beef and cook, breaking it up to combine it with the vegetables and spices, until the meat is brown all the way through, 5 to 8 minutes. Taste to check the seasoning and add more salt and pepper if needed.

Before removing the mixture from the heat, add the lime juice and cilantro and stir to combine.

Serve in butter/Bibb lettuce "cups" with lime wedges and additional garnishes of your choice.

INGREDIENT TIP
*Check out page 224 for a list of recommended brands.

LEFTOVERS MAKEOVER
Use leftovers of the beef mixture in a frittata the next morning. Simply place it in an oven-safe skillet, then pour whisked eggs into the pan. Bake in a 350°F oven for twenty to thirty minutes, or until the eggs are set. ●

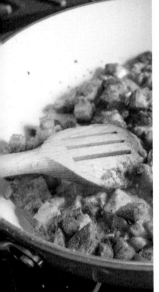

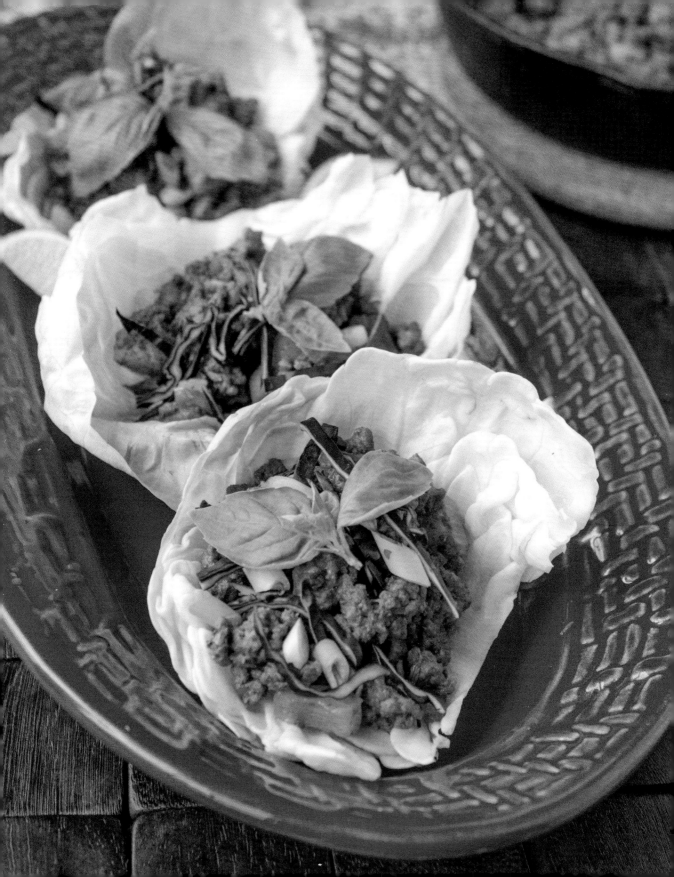

shepherd's pie

PREP TIME **10 MINS** • COOK TIME **50 MINS** • SERVINGS **4-6**

NUTS

EGGS

NIGHTSHADES

FODMAPS

SEAFOOD

1 medium head cauliflower

2 tablespoons unsalted butter, ghee, or other cooking fat

sea salt and black pepper to taste

6 slices bacon, cut into 1/2-inch pieces

3/4 cup diced carrots (approximately 2 large)

2 to 3 cloves garlic, minced or grated

2 pounds ground lamb or beef

1 to 2 fresh sage leaves, minced

1/4 teaspoon ground cinnamon

1 cup peas (thawed if frozen)

NEED MORE CARBS?

Bake 2 or 3 sweet potatoes and mash them up to use as a topping instead of cauliflower. ●

Preheat the oven to 375°F.

Chop the cauliflower roughly into 2-inch pieces. Set up a pot with 1 inch of water and a steamer basket. Steam the cauliflower until fork-tender, approximately 10 minutes. While it's still warm, purée the cauliflower in a food processor with the butter, ghee, or other fat, and season with salt and pepper to taste.

Cook the bacon in a large skillet over medium heat. When the bacon is about halfway done, about 5 minutes, add the diced carrots along with a pinch of salt and pepper. Cook for another few minutes, then add the garlic and ground meat.

When the meat is browned and the carrots are cooked through, add the sage and cinnamon and stir to combine.

Place the meat mixture in an oven-safe baking dish (a pie pan or 9 by 9-inch baking dish works well). Top the meat with a layer of the peas, then a layer of the cauliflower purée. Bake for 20 minutes.

If you wish to brown the top after baking, place the oven rack in the top position, set the broiler to high, and place the dish as close to the heat as possible for 5 to 10 minutes, watching closely to avoid burning it.

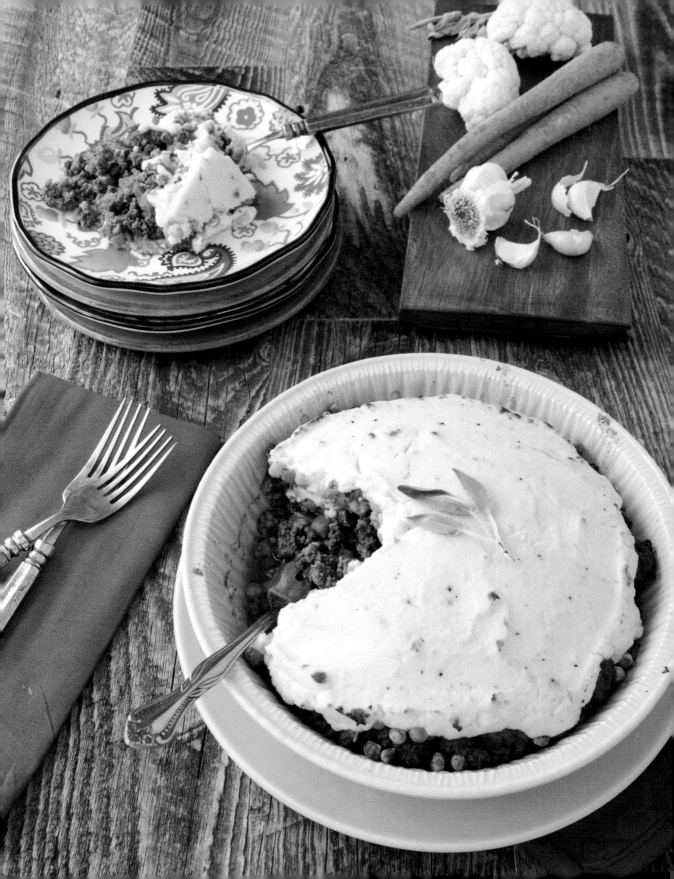

stovetop lamb & chorizo chili

PREP TIME **20 MINS** • COOK TIME **2-3 HRS** • SERVINGS **3-4**

FOR THE CHORIZO

(optional: use 1 pound clean-ingredient, store-bought chorizo)

1 pound ground pork or turkey

2 tablespoons Chorizo Spice Blend (page 208)

1 1/2 tablespoons apple cider vinegar

FOR THE CHILI

1 tablespoon bacon fat, ghee, or coconut oil

1 medium yellow onion, chopped

2 bell peppers, chopped

2 large carrots, chopped

sea salt and black pepper to taste

1 large zucchini, chopped

2 teaspoons minced or grated garlic

1 (14.5-ounce) can diced tomatoes

1 pound ground lamb

2 teaspoons ancho chili powder

1 teaspoon chipotle chili powder (optional)

3 tablespoons chili powder

1 teaspoon ground coriander

2 teaspoons ground cumin

Basic 4 Guacamole (page 185), for serving

USING A SLOW COOKER?

Make the chorizo first, then combine all the ingredients in the slow cooker, set it to low, and cook for approximately 8 hours. ●

Preheat the oven to 425°F.

Make the chorizo: Place the ground meat in a mixing bowl, then sprinkle the Spice Blend evenly over the meat, incorporating it with your hands little by little until all of the Spice Blend is mixed in. Add the vinegar and mix until well combined. Place a quarter of the chorizo in the center of a large sheet of plastic wrap and roll it to form a tightly shaped log—just like you might do to form a log of cookie dough or a sushi roll. When the chorizo is tightly formed, remove it from the plastic wrap and set it on a rimmed baking sheet. Repeat with the remaining meat, creating 3 more logs (4 total). Bake for 25 to 30 minutes. When the chorizo is cool, slice it into 1/4-inch rounds.

Make the chili: In a large enameled cast-iron pot or other non-reactive soup or stew pot, melt the bacon fat, ghee, or coconut oil over medium heat. Add the onion, peppers, and carrots, season with salt and pepper, and cook for about 10 minutes, stirring occasionally, until the vegetables are soft.

Add the zucchini and garlic and stir to combine. Simmer for an additional 5 minutes, then add the diced tomatoes, ground lamb, chili powders, coriander, and cumin, stirring to combine and break up the ground meat into small pieces. Once the ground meat is cooked through, stir in the chorizo.

Simmer the chili over low heat for an additional 1 to 2 hours (depending on how long you have or want to wait) to allow the flavors to meld.

Serve topped with a spoonful of Basic 4 Guacamole.

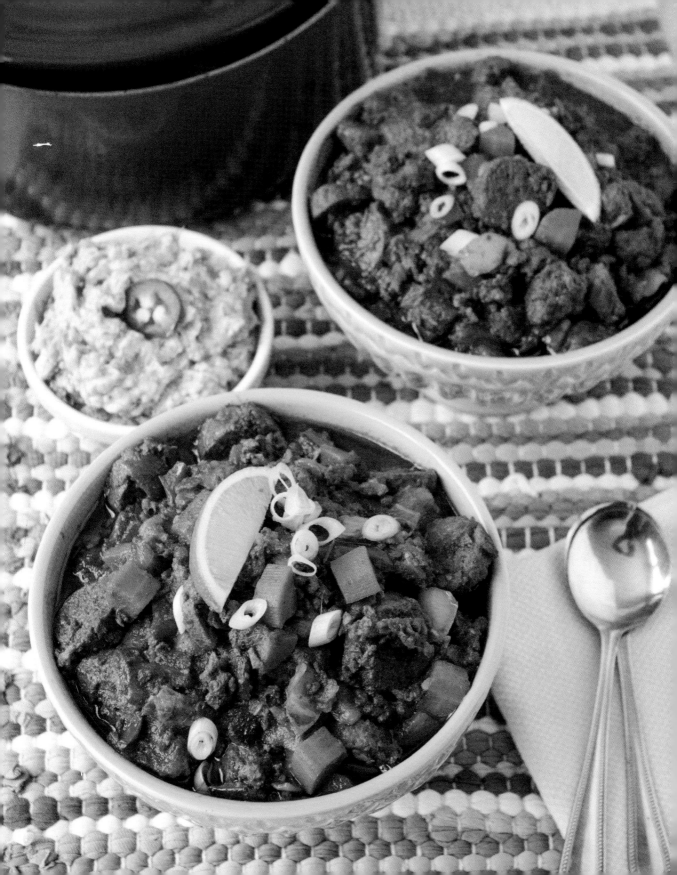

asian-style meatballs

PREP TIME **15 MINS** • COOK TIME **25 MINS** • SERVINGS **4**

NUTS

EGGS

NIGHTSHADES

FODMAPS

SEAFOOD

3 tablespoons coconut aminos*

2 to 3 drops fish sauce (optional)*

1/4 cup sliced green onions (scallions)

1 teaspoon minced or grated garlic

1/2 teaspoon minced fresh ginger

1/2 teaspoon sea salt

1/2 teaspoon black pepper

1 pound ground pork or turkey

1 tablespoon white sesame seeds, for garnish

1 lime, cut into wedges, for garnish

Preheat the oven to 425°F.

In a mixing bowl, combine the coconut aminos, fish sauce (if using), green onions, garlic, ginger, salt, and pepper. Add the meat to the bowl and mix to thoroughly combine with the seasonings. Form the meat into 16 1-ounce meatballs.

Bake for 25 minutes on a rimmed baking sheet. Remove from the oven and garnish with white sesame seeds and lime wedges before serving.

Pictured with Fresh Cabbage & Bok Choy Slaw (page 171).

INGREDIENT TIP
*Check out page 224 for a list of recommended brands. ●

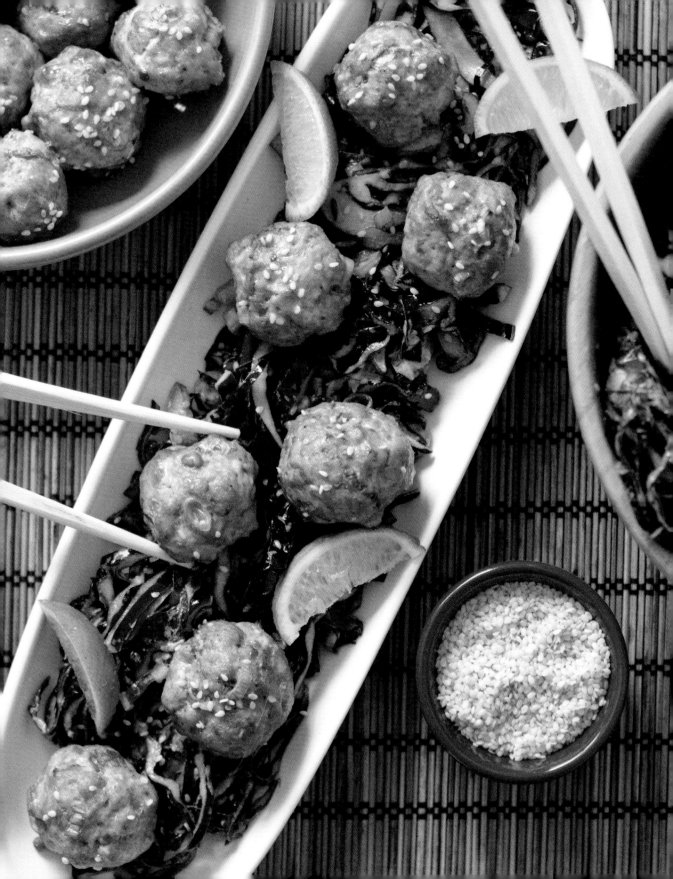

double pork tenderloin

PREP TIME **15 MINS** • COOK TIME **10-15 MINS** • SERVINGS **4**

2 tablespoons Italian Sausage
Spice Blend (page 208)

1 1/2 pounds pork tenderloin
(approximately 2
tenderloins)

10 to 12 slices bacon

FODMAP FREE?
Do not use the Italian
Sausage Spice Blend.
Instead, season the
pork with sage, fennel,
salt, and pepper.

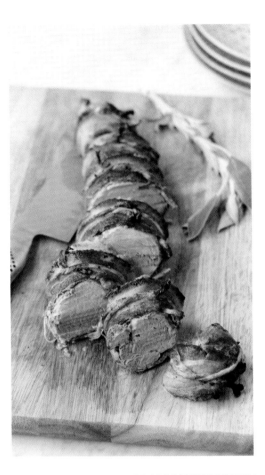

Preheat the oven to 375°F.

Rub the Spice Blend onto the tenderloins, making sure they are evenly covered on all sides. Wrap the slices of bacon around the tenderloins, with the ends meeting underneath.

Cut pieces of cooking twine approximately 6 inches long to match the number of slices of bacon used, then tie a piece around each slice of bacon to hold it in place.

Place a large cast-iron or other oven-safe skillet on the stovetop over medium-high heat. When the pan is hot, sear the tenderloins on all sides until the bacon is browned, approximately 2 minutes per side.

Place the pan in the oven and roast for 10 to 15 minutes or until the internal temperature of the pork reaches at least 145°F.

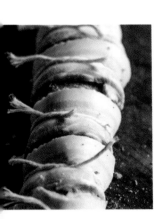

cinnamon grilled pork chops

PREP TIME **5 MINS** • COOK TIME **10-15 MINS** • SERVINGS **4**

- 1/2 teaspoon ground cinnamon
- 1/2 teaspoon granulated garlic
- 1/2 teaspoon sea salt
- 1/2 teaspoon black pepper
- 2 pounds bone-in pork chops, or 1 1/2 pounds boneless chops
- 2 tablespoons bacon fat or coconut oil, melted

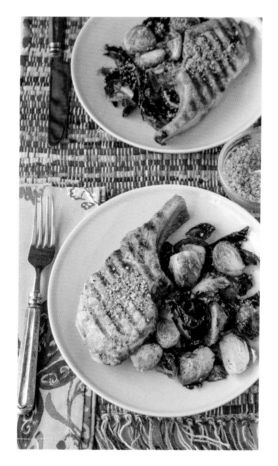

NUTS

EGGS

NIGHTSHADES

FODMAPS

SEAFOOD

Preheat the oven to 400°F.

Heat a large cast-iron or other oven-safe skillet over medium-high heat.

While the skillet heats up, prepare the pork chops: In a small mixing bowl, combine the cinnamon, granulated garlic, salt, and pepper.

Brush the pork chops on both sides with the bacon fat or coconut oil, then sprinkle liberally with the seasoning blend.

Sear the pork chops for approximately 2 to 3 minutes per side (or 1 to 2 minutes if your chops are thin—3/4 inch or less), then transfer the pan to the oven for 5 to 10 minutes or until the internal temperature of the chops reaches at least 145°F. The cooking time will vary with the thickness of the chops—be careful not to overcook thinner cuts.

Pictured with Crumb-Topped Brussels Sprouts (page 181) and a sprinkle of the crumb topping—omit for nut free!

seafood & chorizo paella

PREP TIME **20 MINS** • COOK TIME **60 MINS** • SERVINGS **4**

NUTS

EGGS

NIGHTSHADES

FODMAPS

SEAFOOD

FOR THE CHORIZO

(optional: use 1 pound clean-ingredient, store-bought chorizo)

1 pound ground pork or turkey

2 tablespoons Chorizo Spice Blend (page 208)

1 1/2 tablespoons apple cider vinegar

FOR THE CAULI "RICE"

1 medium head cauliflower (to yield 4 to 5 cups "rice")

1 cup Bone Broth (chicken, page 212)

generous pinch of saffron

1 tablespoon ghee, bacon fat, unsalted butter, or coconut oil

1/2 cup diced red onion

1/2 cup diced orange bell pepper

1/2 cup diced red bell pepper

1 teaspoon minced or grated garlic

12 clams

24 mussels

12 large or jumbo shrimp, peeled and deveined

1/4 cup cooked peas, for garnish (optional)

1 lemon, cut into 4 wedges, for garnish

Make the chorizo: Place the ground meat in a mixing bowl, then sprinkle the Spice Blend evenly over the meat, incorporating it with your hands until all of the Spice Blend is mixed in. Add the vinegar and mix until well combined. Place a quarter of the chorizo in the center of a large sheet of plastic wrap and roll it to form a tightly shaped log—just like you might do to form a log of cookie dough or a sushi roll. Remove it from the plastic wrap and set on a rimmed baking sheet. Repeat with the remaining meat, creating 3 more logs (4 total). Bake for 25 to 30 minutes. When the chorizo is cool, slice it into rounds and set it aside.

Make the cauliflower rice: Chop the cauliflower into florets, then shred or pulse it in a food processor. Set the cauliflower aside. (If you don't have a food processor, you can grate the cauliflower by hand. To do this, quarter the cauliflower head and use a box grater.)

Steep the saffron: In a small saucepan, warm the chicken broth over medium heat, then place the saffron in the broth and allow it to steep for approximately 10 minutes, turning the broth a rich orange color.

Melt the ghee in an extra-large skillet or enameled cast-iron sauté pan or paella pan over medium heat. Sauté the onion and bell peppers until the onion is translucent and just beginning to brown slightly, approximately 5 minutes. Add the garlic and stir to combine, then add the saffron broth.

Add the shredded cauliflower to the pan with the onions, peppers, and garlic; stir to combine. Reduce the heat to medium-low, add the shrimp, and simmer for approximately 5-6 minutes, stirring occasionally until the shrimp is pink all the way through and the cauliflower is cooked through but not mushy.

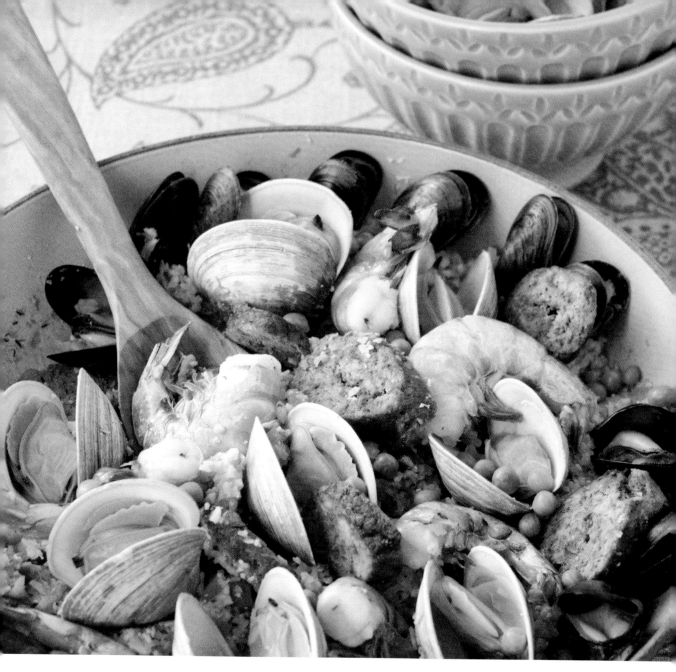

While the "rice" simmers, prepare the shellfish: Fill a large pot with 1 inch of water and bring to a boil, covered, over high heat. Place the clams in the bottom, then the mussels on top of the clams. Allow the shellfish to steam until they open, then remove them and arrange them in the pan with the finished cauliflower "rice." (The mussels will take approximately 5 minutes to open; the clams, 10 to 12 minutes.)

Arrange the sliced chorizo in the pan with the cauliflower "rice" and seafood, then garnish with the peas, if using, and lemon wedges. Serve any shellfish that doesn't fit in the pan alongside the dish to be added to each person's plate after serving a portion from the pan.

spicy sesame-lime salmon

PREP TIME **5 MINS** • COOK TIME **10-12 MINS** • SERVINGS **4**

NUTS

EGGS

NIGHTSHADES

FODMAPS

SEAFOOD

2 tablespoons ghee or coconut oil, melted

4 (4- to 6-ounce) wild salmon fillets

4 tablespoons Spicy Sesame Ginger Dressing (page 216)

2 tablespoons white sesame seeds

1 lime, cut into wedges

1 tablespoon red chili flakes (optional)

KITCHEN TIP

Fish is one of the easiest proteins to cook, despite the rampant fear folks seem to have around preparing it! The keys to making tasty fish recipes at home are as follows: 1) Keep it simple—using basic seasoning and some lemon usually yields the best results; 2) cook it less than you think you need to—most fish cooks in well under 15 minutes, so it's a perfect weeknight protein; and 3) buy it as fresh as you can afford—most people who've said they don't like the fishy taste of fish have always eaten frozen or previously frozen fish. Buying fresh, wild-caught fish that's on sale where you shop and cooking it that night will keep your fish tasting great and not super fishy! ●

Preheat the oven to 350°F.

Brush an oven-safe pan with the ghee or coconut oil in the shape of your pieces of fish, then place the salmon in the pan on the greased areas.

Brush each piece of fish with 1 tablespoon of the Spicy Sesame Ginger Dressing, then sprinkle each piece with 1/2 tablespoon of the white sesame seeds.

Bake for 10 to 12 minutes or until the fish is light pink all the way through.

Squeeze a lime wedge over each piece of fish and sprinkle with chili flakes, if using.

Pictured with Cucumber Cold Noodle Salad (page 170).

lemon sole with almonds & thyme

PREP TIME **5 MINS** • COOK TIME **8-10 MINS** • SERVINGS **4**

2 tablespoons coconut oil or unsalted butter, melted

2 pounds lemon sole or other delicate white fish fillets

sea salt and black pepper to taste

1 lemon, halved

1/4 cup sliced almonds

3 to 5 sprigs fresh thyme

NUTS

EGGS

NIGHTSHADES

FODMAPS

SEAFOOD

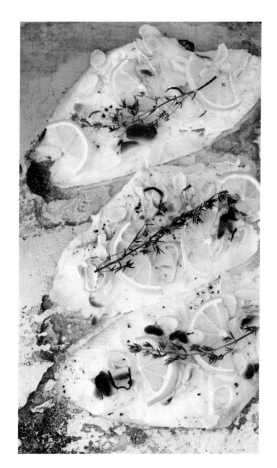

Place the oven rack in the top position and preheat the broiler to high.

Brush a rimmed baking sheet generously with the coconut oil or butter, then place the fish in the pan and brush the tops of the fish as well.

Liberally season both sides of the fish with salt and pepper. Squeeze the juice of half of the lemon over the fish, then sprinkle the sliced almonds evenly on top. Thinly slice the other half of the lemon, then cut the slices in half into half-moons and arrange them on top of the almonds.

Place the thyme sprigs on top of the fish and place the pan in the oven. Broil for 8 to 10 minutes, depending on thickness, until the fish is opaque all the way through.

broiled salmon with caper & olive tapenade

PREP TIME **10 MINS** • COOK TIME **10-12 MINS** • SERVINGS **4**

NUTS

EGGS

NIGHTSHADES

FODMAPS

SEAFOOD

1 tablespoon ghee or coconut oil, melted

4 (4- to 6-ounce) wild salmon fillets

sea salt and black pepper to taste

1 lemon, zested and juiced, divided

1/2 cup capers, drained

1/2 cup pitted kalamata olives

1/4 cup extra-virgin olive oil

1/2 teaspoon dried oregano

1/2 cup cherry tomatoes, quartered

CHEF NOTE
If your oven or toaster oven does not have a broil setting, you can bake the salmon at 350°F for 10 to 12 minutes.

NIGHTSHADE FREE?
Omit the tomatoes.

ON THE SIDE
Serve this salmon with steamed green beans or another green vegetable topped with sliced olives, lemon zest, and a drizzle of extra-virgin olive oil. ●

Place the oven rack in the top position and preheat the broiler to low.

Line a large baking pan with foil. Brush the foil with the ghee or coconut oil in the shape of your pieces of fish. Place the salmon on the greased portions of the foil, season liberally with salt and pepper, and top with half of the lemon zest and lemon juice.

Broil for 10 to 12 minutes or until the fish is light pink all the way through.

While the salmon broils, combine the capers, olives, olive oil, the remaining lemon zest and juice, oregano, and a few pinches each of salt and pepper in a small food processor and pulse just a few times to combine. Set the mixture aside.

When the salmon is cooked, remove it from the oven and plate it topped with the caper and olive tapenade as well as the cherry tomato pieces.

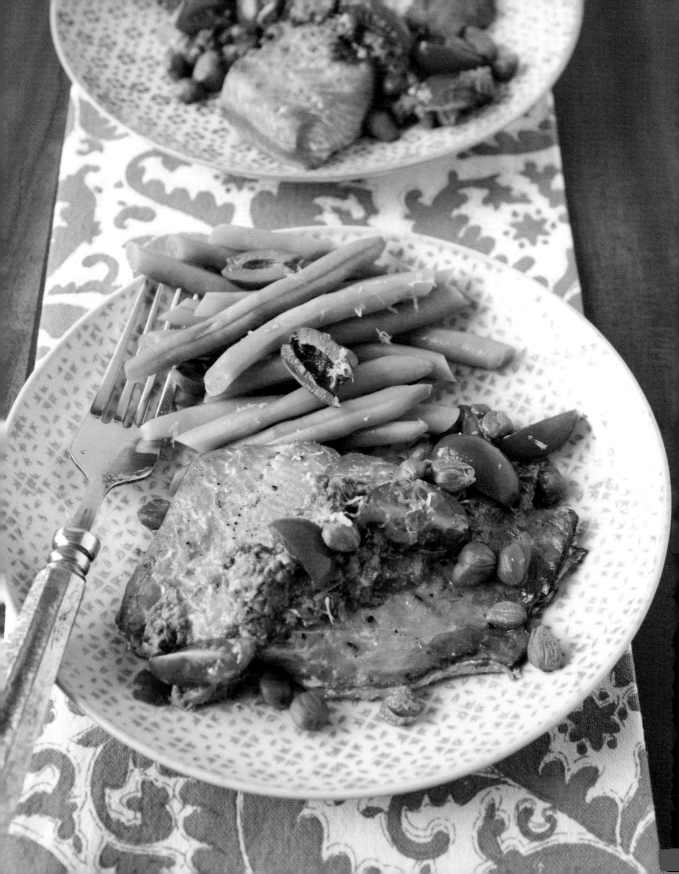

shrimp pad thai

PREP TIME **15 MINS** • COOK TIME **10 MINS** • SERVINGS **4**

4 large zucchini or yellow squash

1 cup snow peas, sliced lengthwise into thin strips

4 dozen extra-large shrimp, peeled and deveined

FOR THE SAUCE

1/2 cup almond butter (raw or roasted)*

1/2 cup coconut aminos*

4 drops fish sauce*

1/2 teaspoon minced or grated garlic

1/4 teaspoon minced fresh ginger

sea salt and black pepper to taste

FOR GARNISH

1 tablespoon white sesame seeds

1/4 cup sliced green onions (scallions)

1/4 cup thinly sliced cucumber

Fill a large pot with 1 inch of water and bring to a boil, covered, over high heat. Place a steamer basket in the pot.

While the water comes to a boil, shred the zucchini or yellow squash into noodles using a handheld julienne peeler, a spiralizer tool, or even a regular vegetable peeler (if using a regular peeler, the noodles will be wide and flat versus spaghetti shaped). You should get 4 cups of noodles. When the water is boiling, steam the noodles in the basket for 3 minutes, then remove them and set them in a colander to drain off the excess liquid as they cool slightly. Place the snow peas on top of the noodles in the colander.

Place the shrimp in the steamer basket over the still-boiling water and cook for 4 to 5 minutes or until pink all the way through. The cooking time will vary with the size of the shrimp.

In a small mixing bowl, whisk together the sauce ingredients until well combined.

Place the noodles, snow peas, sauce, and shrimp in a large skillet over medium-high heat; toss gently to combine and heat through.

To serve, garnish with sesame seeds and top with the green onion and cucumber slices.

INGREDIENT TIP

*Check out page 224 for a list of recommended brands.

KITCHEN TIP

Making zucchini noodles is easy with the right tools. Check out The 21-Day Sugar Detox shop for my favorite picks: balancedbites.com/21dsd ●

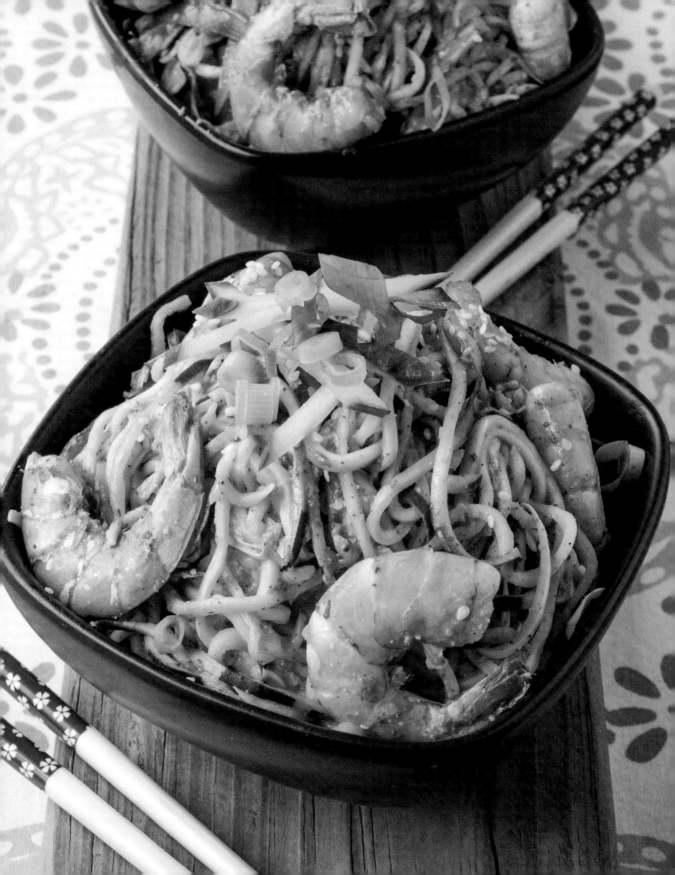

rainbow collard wraps with herb almond "cheese" spread

PREP TIME **20 MINS** • SERVINGS **4**

NUTS

EGGS

NIGHTSHADES

FODMAPS

SEAFOOD

1 cup Herb Almond "Cheese" Spread (page 182)

8 large collard greens

1 pound thinly sliced turkey or chicken breast*

1/2 cup thinly sliced red bell pepper

1/2 cup shredded red cabbage

1/2 cup grated beets

1/2 cup grated carrots

1/4 cup thinly sliced green onions (scallions)

If you do not have 1 cup of leftover Herb Almond "Cheese" Spread on hand, make a new batch. The almonds require 8 hours of soaking time, so be sure to factor in this time when making these wraps.

Lay the collard greens flat on a cutting board and remove the stems, keeping the leaves connected at the top.

Overlap the greens so there is no space between the sides. On each leaf, lay 2 to 3 slices of turkey or chicken, then spread 2 tablespoons of the Herb Almond "Cheese" Spread over the meat. Layer the vegetables on top.

Wrap each collard leaf like a burrito, folding the bottom up first, then the sides, then continuing to roll until all the contents are tucked inside.

Wrap in plastic and store in the refrigerator until mealtime, serving 2 wraps per person.

INGREDIENT TIP
*Check out page 224 for a list of recommended brands.

NIGHTSHADE FREE?
Leave the bell peppers out of the veggie mix inside the wraps. ●

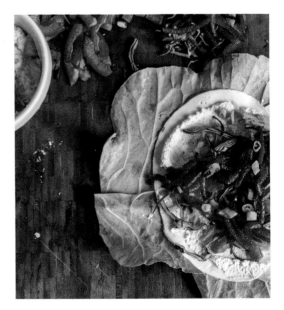

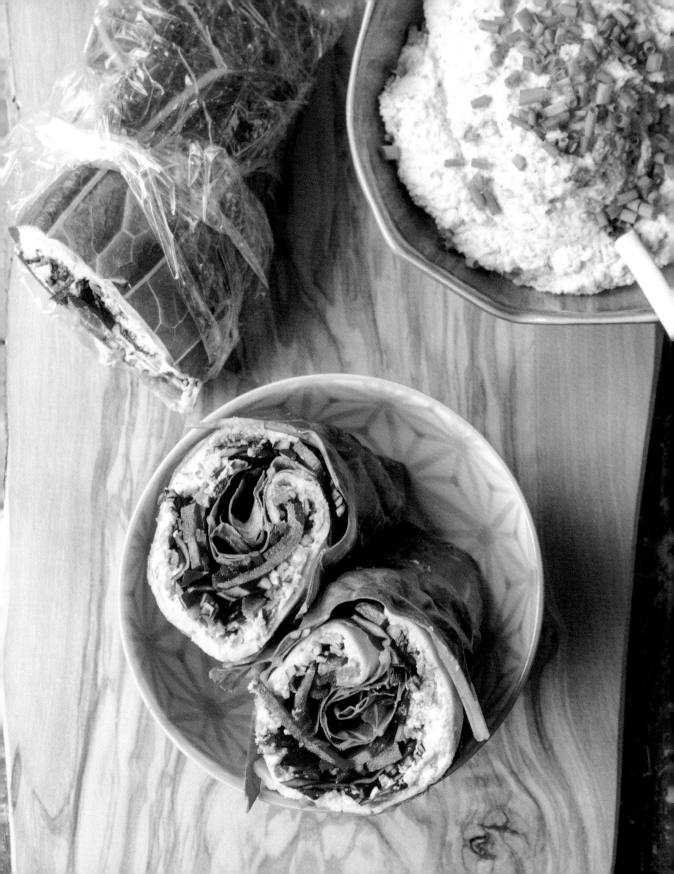

tuna salad wraps

PREP TIME **15 MINS** • SERVINGS **4**

NUTS

EGGS

NIGHTSHADES

FODMAPS

SEAFOOD

4 (6-ounce) cans tuna

1/2 cup Healthy Homemade Mayonnaise (page 211)

1/2 cup minced celery

1 green apple, minced

1/4 cup kelp flakes or minced nori* (dried seaweed paper)

sea salt and black pepper to taste

12 to 16 large lettuce leaves or other raw greens such as collards or kale, stems removed

1/2 cup sliced green onions (scallions), for garnish (optional)

In a food processor, pulse the tuna with the mayonnaise until it's a creamy texture.

Transfer the tuna to a mixing bowl and add the celery, apple, and kelp flakes or nori. Using a large spoon or spatula, mix the salad ingredients until well combined. Season with salt and pepper.

Fill the lettuce leaves or greens of your choice with equal amounts of the tuna salad and garnish with the sliced green onions, if using.

INGREDIENT TIP
*Check out page 224 for a list of recommended brands.

EGG FREE?
Use extra-virgin olive oil instead of mayonnaise to add fat to the fish. Start with 1/4 cup, drizzling it in as the food processor is running. Taste and drizzle in more if needed. ●

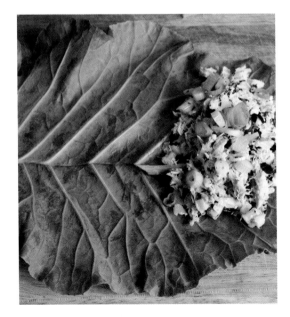

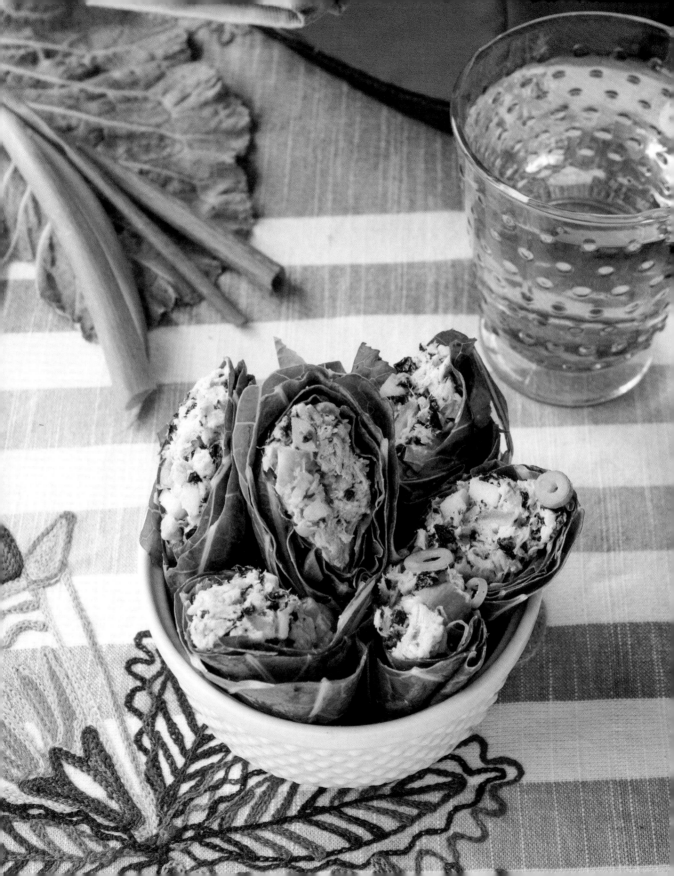

salmon salad with capers & tomato

PREP TIME **15 MINS** • SERVINGS **6**

NUTS

EGGS

NIGHTSHADES

FODMAPS

SEAFOOD

4 (6-ounce) cans salmon*

1/2 cup Healthy Homemade Mayonnaise (page 211)

1 cup diced tomatoes

1/4 cup capers, drained

juice of 1 lemon

sea salt and black pepper to taste

lettuce leaves, for serving (optional)

In a food processor, pulse the salmon with the mayonnaise until it's creamy in texture.

Transfer the salmon to a mixing bowl and add the tomatoes, capers, and lemon juice. Mix to combine, then season with salt and pepper.

Enjoy this salad wrapped in lettuce leaves or served over salad greens—or straight up with a fork!

INGREDIENT TIP
*Check out page 224 for a list of recommended brands.

EGG FREE?
Use extra-virgin olive oil instead of mayonnaise to add fat to the fish. Start with 1/4 cup, drizzling it in as the food processor is running. Taste and drizzle in more if needed. ●

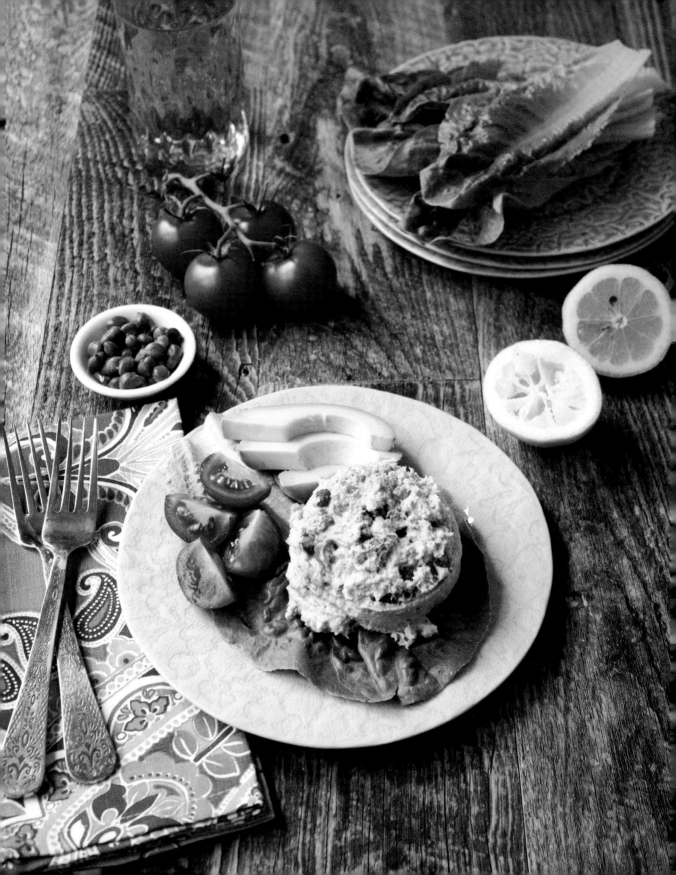

buffalo shrimp lettuce cups

PREP TIME **20 MINS** • COOK TIME **10 MINS** • SERVINGS **4**

NUTS

EGGS

NIGHTSHADES

FODMAPS

SEAFOOD

4 dozen medium shrimp, peeled and deveined

1/4 cup hot sauce*

1/4 cup coconut oil or unsalted butter, melted

2 tablespoons fresh lemon juice

sea salt and black pepper to taste

1-2 heads lettuce of your choice, separated into leaves

1 to 2 avocados, sliced

INGREDIENT TIP
*Check out page 224 for a list of recommended brands. ●

Set up a pot with 1 inch of water and a steamer basket. Bring to a boil, covered, over high heat. Steam the shrimp for approximately 5 minutes until pink and white all the way through. You may need to cook it in 2 batches to avoid crowding your steamer basket.

While they're warm, chop the shrimp into bite-sized pieces.

In a mixing bowl, whisk together the hot sauce, coconut oil or butter, and lemon juice.

Toss the shrimp in the hot sauce mixture, season with salt and pepper, and serve in lettuce wraps topped with avocado slices.

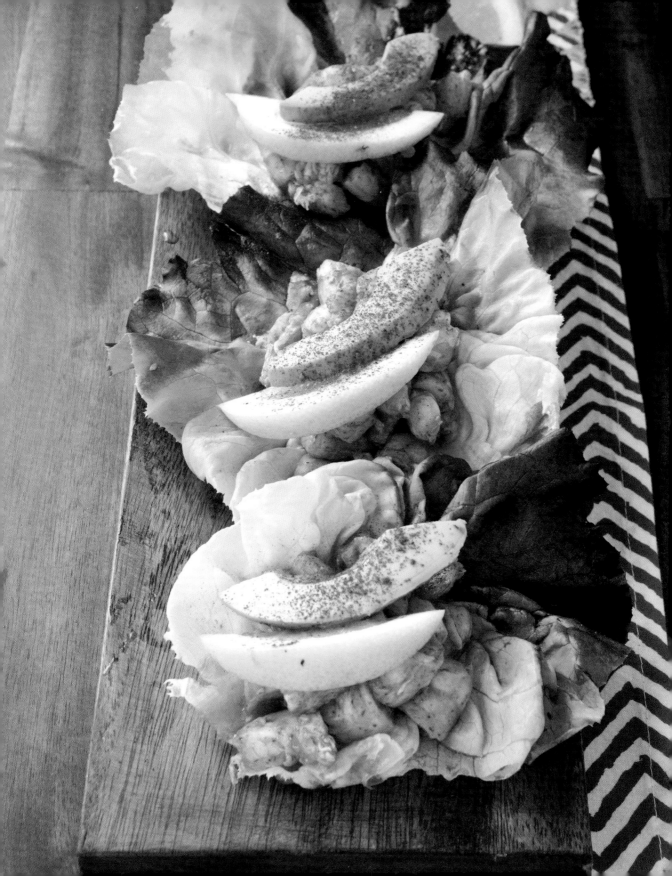

smoky chicken tortilla-less soup

PREP TIME **30 MINS** • COOK TIME **45 MINS** • SERVINGS **4**

NUTS

EGGS

NIGHTSHADES

FODMAPS

SEAFOOD

2 tablespoons coconut oil or bacon fat

1 small onion, diced

1 red bell pepper, diced

2 carrots, diced

2 stalks celery, diced

1 poblano pepper, roasted, peeled, and diced (see Kitchen Tip)

sea salt and black pepper to taste

2 teaspoons ground cumin

2 teaspoons ground coriander

1/2 teaspoon chipotle powder

7 ounces tomato paste

1 quart Bone Broth (chicken or beef, page 212)

1/2 pound boneless, skinless chicken, cooked and shredded

OPTIONAL GARNISHES

1/4 cup chopped fresh cilantro leaves

1 avocado, sliced

In a large soup pot, melt the coconut oil or bacon fat over medium heat. Put the onion in the pot and cook until it becomes translucent and the edges begin to brown. Add the bell pepper, carrots, celery, roasted poblano pepper, salt, and pepper to taste. Add the cumin, coriander, and chipotle powder and stir until well combined. Cook for a few more minutes until the vegetables are soft.

Stir in the tomato paste and Bone Broth and season with salt and pepper again if needed. Reduce the heat to low and simmer for 20 minutes or until the flavors are well combined. When the soup is nearly done, add the cooked chicken to the pot just to heat it all the way through. Taste once more and adjust the seasoning if needed.

Serve garnished with the cilantro and avocado slices, if desired.

KITCHEN TIP

To roast the poblano pepper, simply place the whole pepper over a low, open gas flame directly on the grate, turning regularly with tongs until the skin is blackened on all sides. Place the pepper in a bowl, cover, and set aside for few minutes. Then gently remove the blackened skin with your hands. If the pepper is still very hot to the touch, you may run it under some warm water while you remove the blackened skin, but this may weaken the flavor of the pepper slightly, so waiting for it to cool just enough to handle is ideal. Use the seeds if you like; poblanos aren't known for being super hot. ●

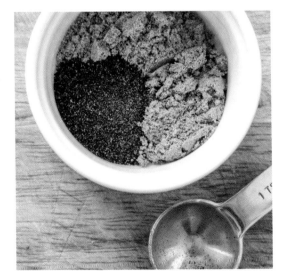

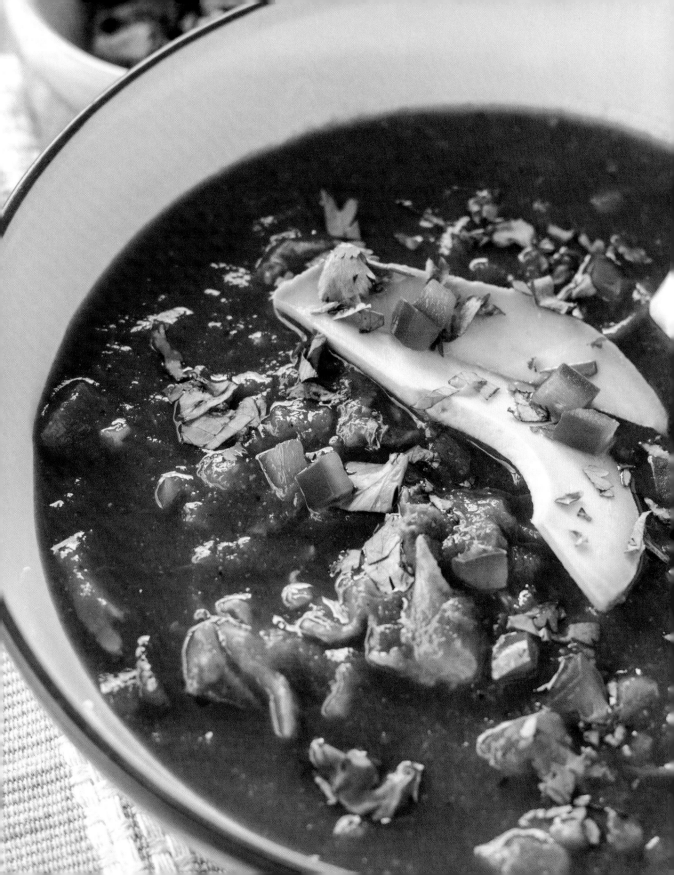

roasted cauliflower soup

PREP TIME 15 MINS • COOK TIME 45 MINS • SERVINGS 4

NUTS

EGGS

NIGHTSHADES

FODMAPS

SEAFOOD

1 medium head cauliflower

3 tablespoons ghee,
bacon fat, or coconut oil,
divided

sea salt and black pepper
to taste

1/2 cup diced onion

1/2 cup diced carrot

1 teaspoon fresh rosemary
or other fresh herbs of
your choice

3 cups Bone Broth
(chicken, page 212)

OPTIONAL GARNISHES

4 teaspoons extra-virgin
olive oil or truffle oil

2 slices bacon, cooked and
diced

Preheat the oven to 375°F.

Chop the cauliflower into 1- to 2-inch pieces. Place the cauliflower in a large roasting pan. Melt 2 tablespoons of the ghee, bacon fat, or coconut oil and drizzle it over the cauliflower. Toss the cauliflower to evenly coat and season liberally with salt and pepper. Roast the cauliflower for 30 to 40 minutes or until the edges begin to brown.

While the cauliflower roasts, prepare the rest of the soup ingredients. Melt the remaining 1 tablespoon ghee, bacon fat, or coconut oil in a soup pot over medium heat and sauté the onion, carrot, and rosemary along with a dash of salt and pepper until the onions are translucent and the carrots are soft, approximately 8 minutes. Add the Bone Broth, reduce the heat to low, and simmer for 10 minutes.

Reserve 1/2 to 1 cup of the roasted cauliflower for garnish. Place 2 cups of the roasted cauliflower plus 2 cups of the broth mixture in a blender—taking care not to fill it too much, as hot liquids tend to expand in the blender. Put the blender lid firmly in place on top of the pitcher, but remove the center "valve" piece from the lid. Hold a thick kitchen towel over the lid, covering the hole where the valve normally stays. Blend on low at first, then briefly blend on high. This will give your soup a creamy texture. You may choose to blend all the cauliflower and broth mixture; if so, do it in batches so as not to overfill your blender.

Add the blended soup back to the soup pot and stir to combine. Serve garnished with the reserved roasted cauliflower chunks and a drizzle of a high-quality extra-virgin olive oil or truffle oil and/or chopped bacon, if using.

KITCHEN TIP

Cauliflower not your favorite? Make this recipe using carrots instead of cauliflower.

NEED MORE CARBS?

Use butternut squash instead of cauliflower. ●

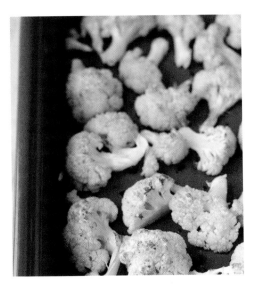

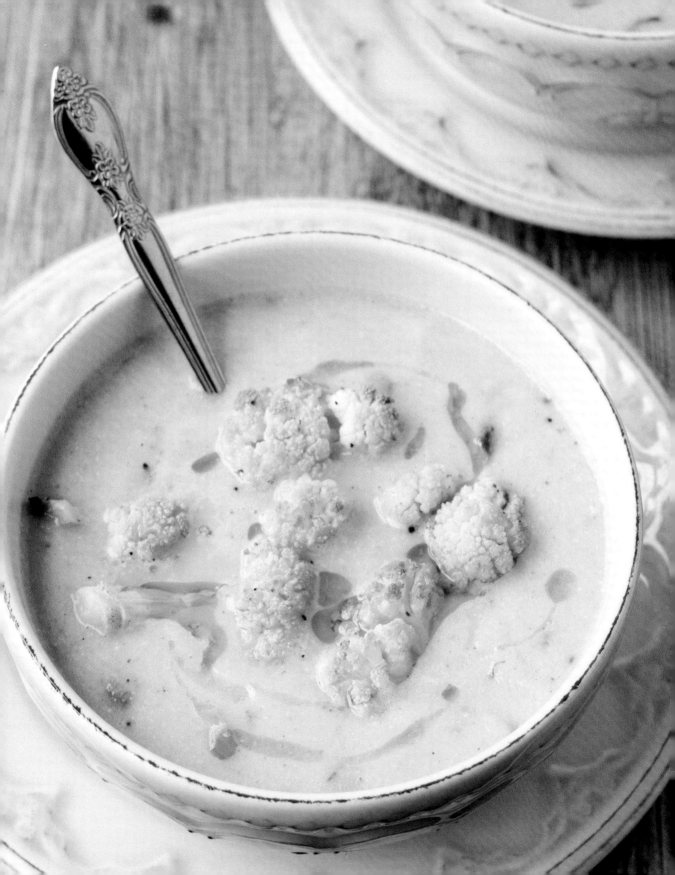

simple spinach & garlic soup

PREP TIME 5 MINS • COOK TIME 10 MINS • SERVINGS 4

1 tablespoon ghee or coconut oil

2 to 3 cloves garlic, smashed

3 cups Bone Broth (chicken, page 212)

3 cups packed spinach

1 avocado, halved

sea salt and black pepper to taste

OPTIONAL GARNISHES

1/4 cup full-fat coconut milk*

2 tablespoons minced fresh chives

INGREDIENT TIP

*Check out page 224 for a list of recommended brands.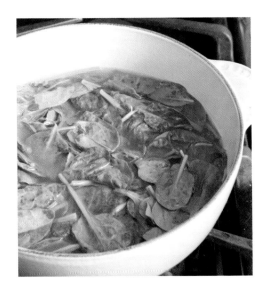

In a soup pot, melt the ghee or coconut oil over medium heat. Place the smashed garlic in the pan. When the garlic just begins to brown, add the Bone Broth and bring it to a simmer. Add the spinach to the pot and simmer until wilted, approximately 1 minute.

Transfer the soup to a blender in 2 batches, pouring half of the soup and adding half of the avocado at a time. Put the blender lid firmly in place on top of the pitcher, but remove the center "valve" piece from the lid. Hold a thick kitchen towel over the lid, covering the hole where the valve normally stays. Blend each half of the soup with the avocado, then recombine in the original pot and whisk the mixture together. Season to taste with salt and pepper.

Serve 1 cup of soup per person, garnishing each serving with 1 tablespoon of the coconut milk and 1/2 tablespoon of the chives, if using.

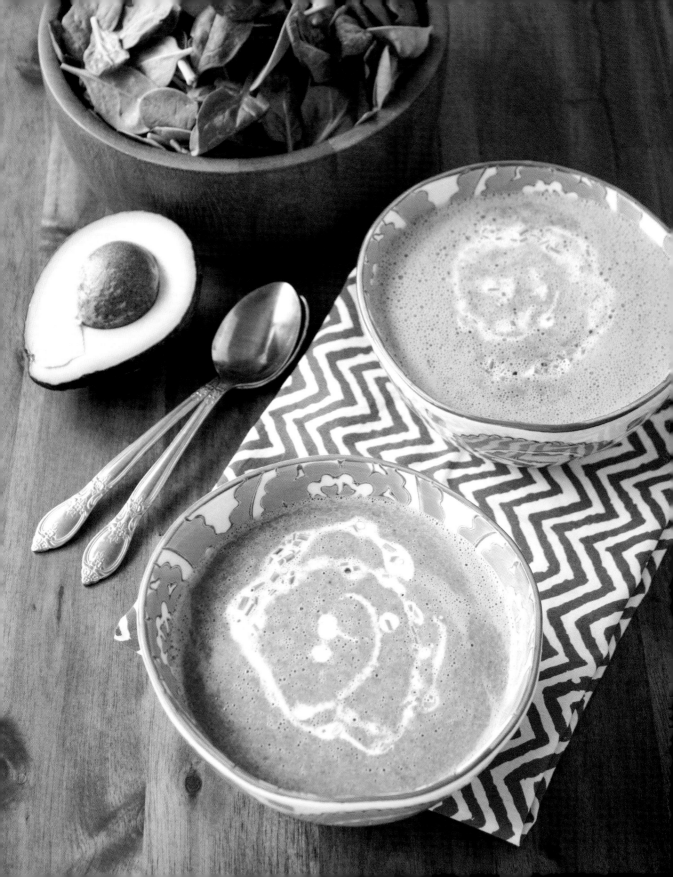

no-miso soup

PREP TIME 10 MINS • COOK TIME 10 MINS • SERVINGS 4

NUTS

EGGS

NIGHTSHADES

FODMAPS

SEAFOOD

32 ounces Bone Broth
(chicken, page 212)

2 tablespoons coconut
aminos*

3 drops fish sauce*

1 cup sliced baby bok choy
(about 2 bulbs)

8 ounces cooked shrimp,
chopped (optional; not
pictured)

2 green onions (scallions),
sliced

sea salt and black pepper
to taste

1/4 cup chopped fresh
cilantro leaves, for
garnish

Simmer the Bone Broth, coconut aminos, and
fish sauce in a saucepan over medium-low heat
for about 10 minutes or until it comes to a low
boil.

Add the bok choy and green onions and
simmer for an additional 2 to 3 minutes until
the bok choy becomes bright green and
softens. *If you are adding cooked shrimp to this
soup, add it with the bok choy to heat through.*
Season with salt and pepper to taste.

Garnish with cilantro.

INGREDIENT TIP
*Check out page
224 for a list of
recommended
brands

SEAFOOD FREE?
Omit the fish
sauce.

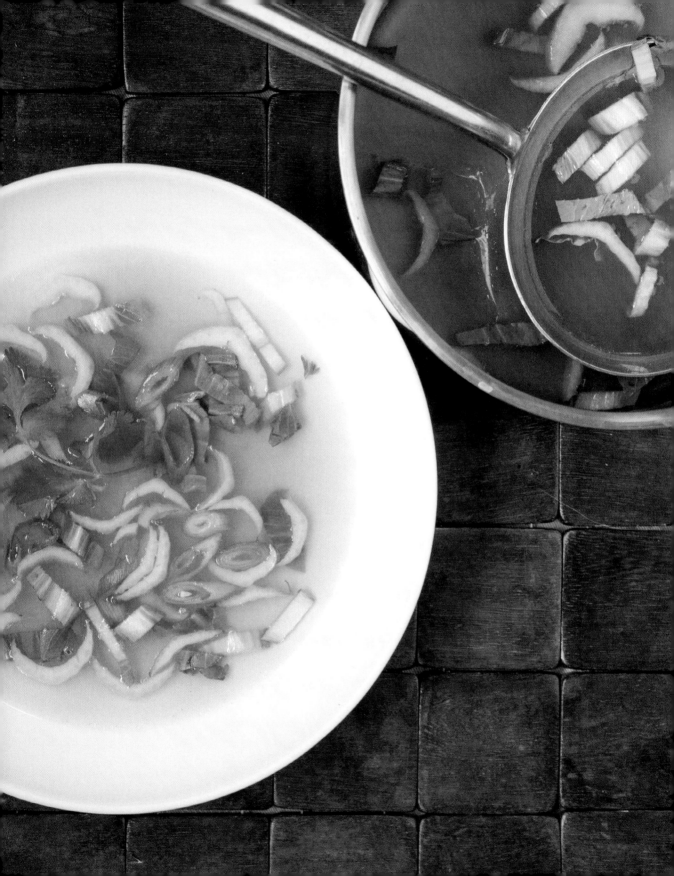

seared tuna, grapefruit, & asparagus salad

PREP TIME 15 MINS • COOK TIME 5 MINS • SERVINGS 5

NUTS

EGGS

NIGHTSHADES

FODMAPS

SEAFOOD

FOR THE TUNA

1 to 1 1/2 pounds wild tuna steaks

sea salt and black pepper to taste

1 lime, halved

2 tablespoons white sesame seeds

1 tablespoon coconut oil

FOR THE DRESSING

1/4 cup macadamia nut oil or cold-pressed sesame seed oil

juice of 1 lime

2 tablespoons minced shallot

2 tablespoons minced fresh cilantro leaves

sea salt and black pepper to taste

FOR THE SALAD

1 large bunch slender asparagus (about 1 1/2 pounds)

2 avocados, sliced

1 ruby red grapefruit, segmented (see Kitchen Tip)

1 teaspoon white sesame seeds, for garnish

Heat an enameled cast-iron or stainless-steel skillet over medium-high heat. Season the tuna steaks with salt and pepper on both sides, then squeeze the lime halves over both sides. Next, sprinkle both sides of the tuna with the sesame seeds to form a thin crust. When the pan is hot, melt the coconut oil, then sear the tuna for 1 minute per side.

In small mixing bowl, whisk together the ingredients for the dressing.

Slice the asparagus into 3 sections each, discarding 1 to 1 1/2 inches of the bottom woody portion. Divide the asparagus among 5 serving plates.

Slice the tuna against the grain into 1/4-inch thick pieces. Place the tuna on top of the asparagus, then top with the avocado slices and grapefruit segments.

Drizzle some of the dressing over each plate and garnish with the sesame seeds.

KITCHEN TIP

To segment your citrus fruit: Using a sharp paring knife, slice along the rounded outer edge of the fruit, carefully removing all of the skin and white pith. Next, carefully slice diagonally from the outside toward the center of the fruit, running the knife next to each thin piece of divider skin to remove the fleshy portions in between. The segments will slide out cleanly and ready to eat!

CHEF NOTE

Yes, asparagus can be eaten raw! If you don't care for it raw after trying it once, you may steam or roast the asparagus before using it in this salad. You may also serve this salad over mixed greens instead of asparagus.

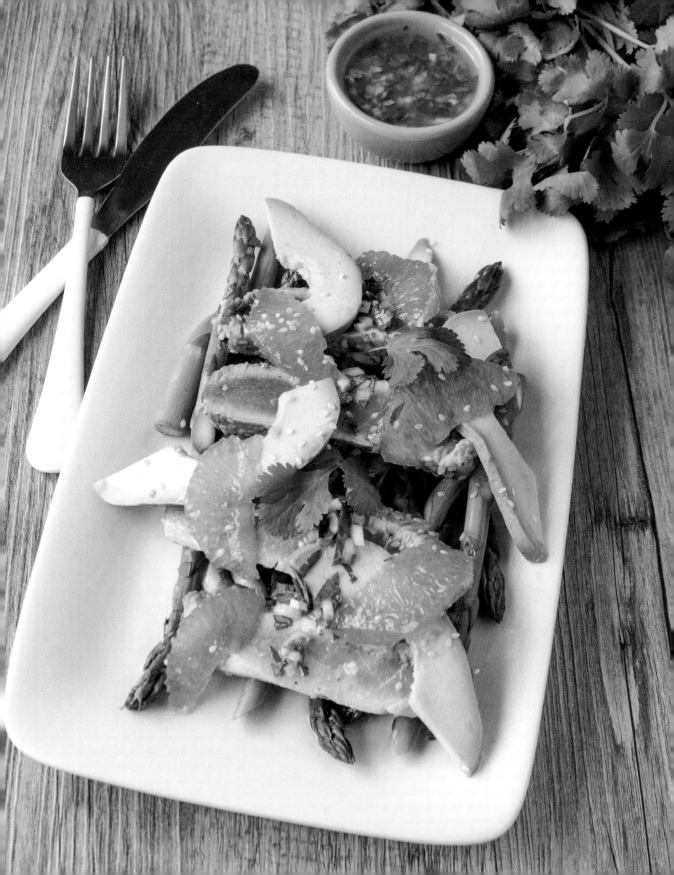

green apple & fennel salad

PREP TIME 10 MINS • SERVINGS 4

NUTS

EGGS

NIGHTSHADES

FODMAPS

SEAFOOD

FOR THE DRESSING

1/2 cup extra-virgin olive oil or macadamia nut oil

2 tablespoons apple cider vinegar

2 tablespoons fresh lemon juice

1/2 teaspoon fennel seeds, ground

1/2 teaspoon ground cinnamon

1/4 teaspoon onion powder

sea salt and black pepper to taste

2 green apples, sliced into matchsticks

1 cup thinly sliced fennel (1 to 2 bulbs)

1/4 teaspoon ground cinnamon, for garnish

Salad greens or baby spinach, for serving (optional; not pictured)

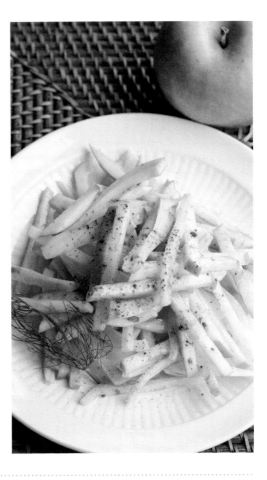

In a small mixing bowl, whisk together all the ingredients for the dressing.

In a medium-sized mixing bowl, toss the dressing with the apples and fennel and garnish with the cinnamon.

Serve alone or over salad greens or baby spinach.

broccoli & bacon salad
with creamy balsamic dressing

PREP TIME 15 MINS • COOK TIME 15 MINS • SERVINGS 4

4 slices bacon

1 large head broccoli

1/4 cup Healthy Homemade Mayonnaise (page 211)

3 tablespoons balsamic vinegar

2 tablespoons minced shallot

sea salt and black pepper to taste

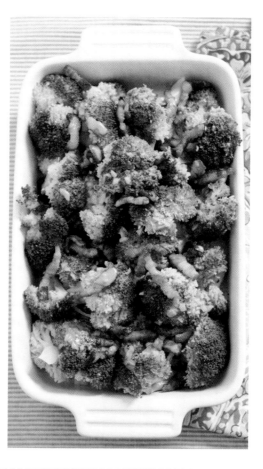

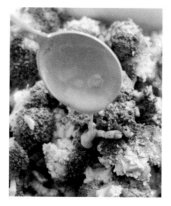

NUTS

EGGS

NIGHTSHADES

FODMAPS

SEAFOOD

EGG FREE?
Use 1/4 cup extra-virgin olive oil plus 1 teaspoon gluten-free Dijon mustard instead of mayonnaise. ●

Slice the bacon crosswise into 1/4-inch strips and cook it in a skillet over medium heat until crispy. Remove the bacon from the pan and set it on paper towels to drain. Reserve the bacon fat for another use.

Chop the broccoli into large florets. Steam the broccoli in a basket over 1 inch of boiling water until it's bright green but not overdone, about 5 minutes. Place the steamed broccoli in a large bowl of ice water to "shock" it—this will keep it from cooking further and maintain its bright color. Drain in a colander.

In a small mixing bowl, whisk together the mayonnaise, vinegar, shallot, salt, and pepper.

In a serving bowl, toss the broccoli with the dressing, then garnish with the bacon strips. Serve at room temperature.

cucumber cold noodle salad

PREP TIME 15 MINS • SERVINGS 4

NUTS

EGGS

NIGHTSHADES

FODMAPS

SEAFOOD

2 large cucumbers

2 tablespoons Spicy Sesame Ginger Dressing (page 216)

2 tablespoons cold-pressed sesame oil

1 tablespoon rice wine vinegar*

1 tablespoon sesame seeds, for garnish

Using a julienne peeler, regular vegetable peeler, or spiralizer tool, cut the cucumber into long, thin "noodles," discarding the seeded part in the center.

In a mixing bowl, toss the cucumber noodles with the Spicy Sesame Ginger Dressing, sesame oil, and vinegar.

Garnish with the sesame seeds and serve chilled or at room temperature.

INGREDIENT TIP
*Check the ingredients and avoid brands that contain added sugar.

SPECIAL EQUIPMENT
You can find julienne peelers or spiralizers easily online or in some local stores. Visit balancedbites.com/21DSD for recommended brands.

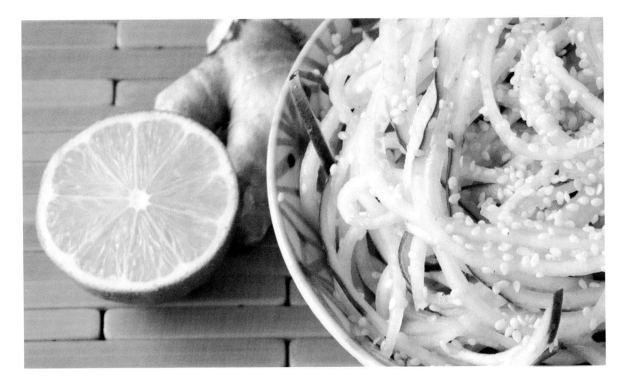

fresh cabbage & bok choy slaw

PREP TIME 15 MINS • SERVINGS 4

2 tablespoons raw tahini (ground sesame paste)

juice of 2 limes

1/4 cup cold-pressed sesame oil

1/4 teaspoon minced or grated garlic

4 cups finely sliced red cabbage (1 medium head)

1 cup finely sliced bok choy

sea salt and black pepper to taste

1/4 cup chopped green onions (scallions), for garnish

1 tablespoon white sesame seeds, for garnish

In a large mixing bowl, whisk together the tahini, lime juice, sesame oil, and garlic. Add the sliced cabbage and boy choy to the bowl and toss to combine. Season with salt and pepper. Garnish with the green onions and sesame seeds.

Serve chilled or at room temperature.

NUTS

EGGS

NIGHTSHADES

FODMAPS

SEAFOOD

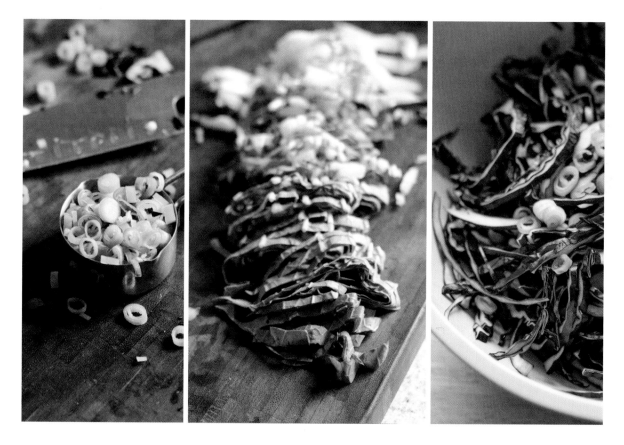

basic cilantro cauli-rice

PREP TIME 15 MINS • COOK TIME 5 MINS • SERVINGS 4

1 head cauliflower

1 tablespoon coconut oil or bacon fat

sea salt and black pepper to taste

1/4 cup finely chopped fresh cilantro leaves

OPTIONAL ADD-INS FOR COLOR & VARIETY

as pictured

1/4 cup minced red onion

1/4 cup minced yellow bell pepper

1 tablespoon coconut oil or bacon fat

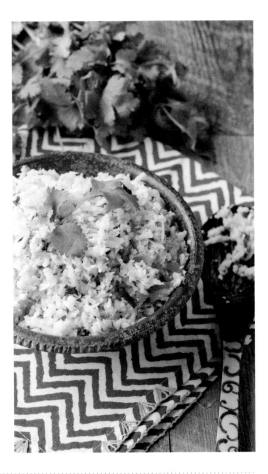

Remove the outer leaves and stem from the cauliflower, and chop it into large chunks. Shred the cauliflower using a box grater or food processor.

If adding red onion and yellow bell pepper, sauté the onion and pepper in the 1 tablespoon of coconut oil or bacon fat in a small skillet over medium heat for about 5 minutes or until they become soft and have golden brown edges.

In a large skillet over medium heat, melt the coconut oil or bacon fat, and place the shredded cauliflower in the skillet. Add salt and pepper to taste. Sauté for about 5 minutes or until the cauliflower begins to become translucent, stirring gently to ensure that it cooks through.

Stir in the optional add-ins (if using), place the cooked cauliflower in a serving bowl, and toss with the chopped cilantro before serving.

balsamic winter squash rings

PREP TIME 5 MINS • COOK TIME 35 MINS • SERVINGS 4

2 kabocha squash (do not peel), or 1 butternut squash, peeled

1/4 cup bacon fat or coconut oil, melted

sea salt and black pepper to taste

1/2 cup balsamic vinegar

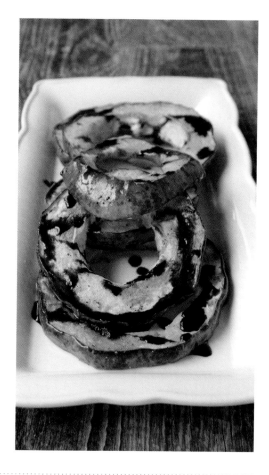

WANT SOME CRUNCH?
Garnish with toasted chopped almonds, macadamia nuts, pecans, or walnuts.

Preheat the oven to 375°F.

Slice the squash into 3/4-inch rings. Remove the seeds with a spoon.

Arrange the squash rings on 2 large rimmed baking sheets and coat evenly with the bacon fat or coconut oil. Season with salt and pepper on both sides. Roast for 20 minutes, then flip the slices and place back in the oven for an additional 15 minutes.

While the squash roasts, heat the balsamic vinegar in a very small saucepan over medium-low heat and allow it to cook down until it becomes slightly thickened and is reduced by about half.

Spoon the balsamic reduction over the roasted squash and serve warm. Note: While you will roast the kabocha squash with the skin on, you can scoop the soft inside from the skin when you eat it.

SOUPS
SALADS
& SIDES

NUTS

EGGS

NIGHTSHADES

FODMAPS

SEAFOOD

jicama fresh "fries"

PREP TIME 5 MINS • SERVINGS 4

1 jicama "bulb"
  (approximately 1 pound)

1 lime or lemon, halved

1/2 to 1 teaspoon chili powder,
  cayenne pepper, or chipotle
  chili powder, to taste

sea salt to taste

**NIGHTSHADE
FREE?**
Omit the chili powder
(or any pepper
powder) and just use
lime or lemon juice
and salt. ●

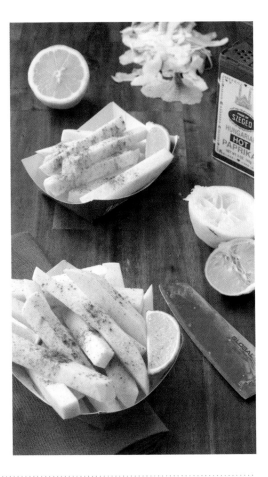

Peel the jicama with a vegetable peeler, then slice it into French fry-sized sticks, approximately 1/4- to 1/2-inch thick.

Place the jicama in a serving bowl and squeeze the lime or lemon halves over the top.

Sprinkle the chili powder or cayenne pepper and salt on top and toss to coat the jicama.

Serve immediately, as the jicama will become soggy if left too long. If you want to make this dish ahead of time, save the lime, chili powder or cayenne pepper, and salt for dressing immediately before eating or serving.

greek tomato & cucumber salad

PREP TIME 10 MINS • SERVINGS 4

2 cups roughly chopped
   tomatoes (heirloom, Roma,
   cherry, etc.—any kind will
   do!)

2 cups roughly chopped
   cucumbers

1/2 cup extra-virgin olive oil

juice of 1 lemon, or 2
   tablespoons balsamic
   vinegar

1 1/2 teaspoons dried oregano

sea salt and black pepper to
   taste

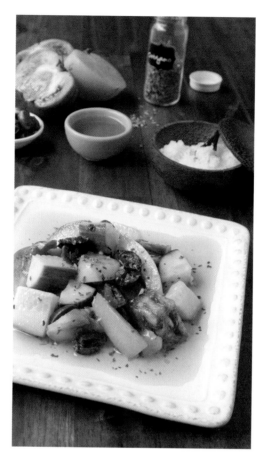

NUTS

EGGS

NIGHTSHADES

FODMAPS

SEAFOOD

**NIGHTSHADE
FREE?**

Make this salad with
just cucumbers, or
replace the tomatoes
with thinly sliced raw
carrot discs.

Toss all ingredients in a large mixing
bowl to combine. Serve cold or at
room temperature.

For even better flavor, allow the
salad to marinate for at least an hour
before serving.

NUTS

EGGS

NIGHTSHADES

FODMAPS

SEAFOOD

lemon & garlic noodles with olives

PREP TIME 15 MINS • COOK TIME 5 MINS • SERVINGS 4

4 large zucchini or yellow squash

sea salt and black pepper to taste

2 tablespoons water

zest and juice of 1 lemon

1/4 cup extra-virgin olive oil

1 clove garlic, minced or grated

1/2 cup pitted kalamata olives, halved

FODMAP FREE?
Omit the garlic.

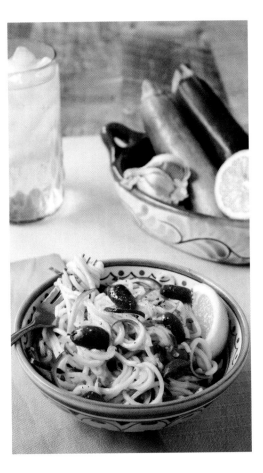

Using a julienne peeler or a spiralizer, cut the zucchini or squash into noodles, with the skin on.

Season the noodles with salt and pepper and place them in a large skillet. Add the water and cook the noodles over medium heat until they're just slightly soft. Place the noodles in a colander and allow them to sit for 5 minutes to drain off the excess water.

Place the lemon zest and juice in a mixing bowl. Whisk in the olive oil and garlic, and add salt and pepper to taste.

Toss the strained noodles with the lemon dressing and olives.

Serve warm or cold.

pesto spaghetti squash

PREP TIME **15 MINS** • COOK TIME **40-50 MINS** • SERVINGS **4**

SOUPS
SALADS
& SIDES

1 spaghetti squash (4 to 5 pounds)

sea salt and black pepper to taste

FOR THE PESTO

1/2 cup shelled pistachios, macadamia nuts, walnuts, pecans, or pine nuts

1 clove garlic

1/2 cup extra-virgin olive oil

sea salt and black pepper to taste

1 bunch fresh cilantro or basil

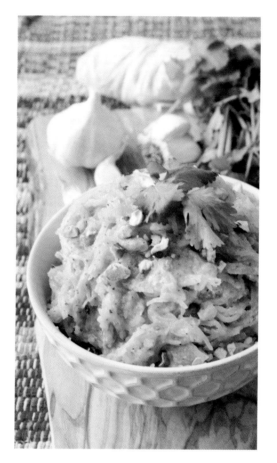

NUTS

EGGS

NIGHTSHADES

FODMAPS

SEAFOOD

Preheat the oven to 375°F.

Cut the spaghetti squash in half lengthwise and remove the seeds and inner membranes, then sprinkle liberally with salt and pepper. Place the squash halves facedown on a baking sheet. Roast for approximately 40 minutes or until the skin gives when you press on it and the "noodles" inside release easily from the skin.

Combine the nuts, garlic, olive oil, salt, and pepper in a food processor, and blend until smooth. Add the cilantro or basil and continue to blend until smooth. Taste for seasoning and add more salt and pepper if needed.

While the squash is warm, use a fork to remove the noodles, then toss with the pesto.

creamy herb mashed cauliflower

PREP TIME 5 MINS • COOK TIME 15 MINS • SERVINGS 4

NUTS

EGGS

NIGHTSHADES

FODMAPS

SEAFOOD

1 large head cauliflower

2 tablespoons unsalted butter or coconut oil

2 tablespoons extra-virgin olive oil

1/2 teaspoon fresh rosemary, or up to 1 teaspoon other fresh herb of your choice

sea salt and black pepper to taste

Cut the cauliflower into 2- to 3-inch pieces. Set up a pot with 1 inch of water and a steamer basket. Bring to a boil, covered, over high heat. Steam the cauliflower until it is fork-tender, then place it in a food processor along with the butter or coconut oil, olive oil, rosemary or other herb, salt, and pepper. Purée until smooth and creamy.

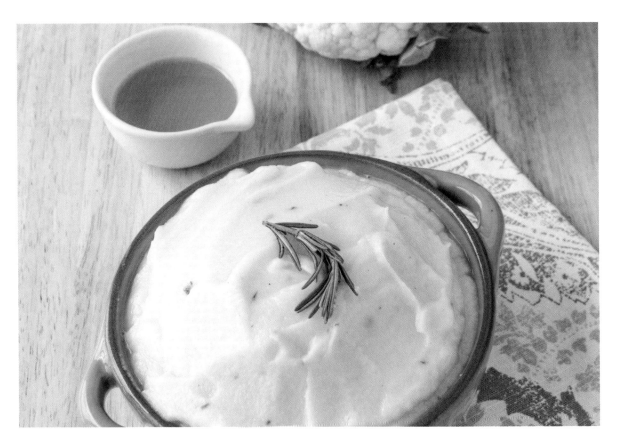

cocoa-chili roasted cauliflower

PREP TIME 10 MINS • COOK TIME 30 MINS • SERVINGS 4

2 medium heads cauliflower

1/4 cup coconut oil, melted

1/2 teaspoon unsweetened cocoa powder*

1/2 teaspoon chili powder

1/2 teaspoon ground cinnamon

1/2 teaspoon onion powder

1/2 teaspoon sea salt

1/2 teaspoon black pepper

NUTS

EGGS

NIGHTSHADES

FODMAPS

SEAFOOD

INGREDIENT TIP
*Check out page 224 for a list of recommended brands. ●

Preheat the oven to 425°F.

Chop the cauliflower into 1/4- to 1/2-inch pieces. In a large mixing bowl, gently toss the cauliflower with the coconut oil.

In a small mixing bowl, combine the cocoa powder, chili powder, cinnamon, onion powder, salt, and pepper. Sprinkle the spice mixture evenly over the cauliflower and toss gently with your hands, massaging the oil and spices into the cauliflower.

Spread the cauliflower evenly in a single layer on 2 rimmed baking sheets and roast for 30 minutes, until tender and starting to caramelize.

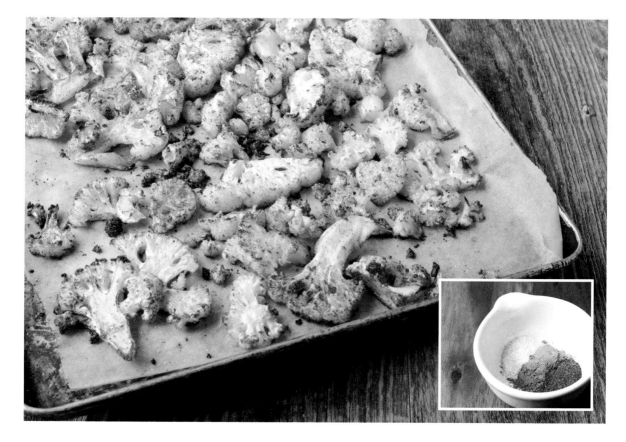

NUTS

EGGS

NIGHTSHADES

FODMAPS

SEAFOOD

golden beets with crispy herbs

PREP TIME 5 MINS • COOK TIME 30-35 MINS • SERVINGS 4

3-4 medium golden beets

3 tablespoons bacon fat or coconut oil, divided

1/4 teaspoon sea salt

1/4 teaspoon black pepper

2 sprigs fresh rosemary

10-12 fresh sage leaves

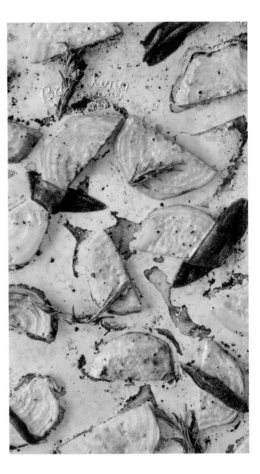

Preheat the oven to 425°F.

Slice the tops off of the beets and peel off the outer skins. Slice the beets in half lengthwise, then into 1/4-inch half-moons.

Toss the beets with 1 tablespoon of the bacon fat or coconut oil and season with the salt and pepper. Roast in a single layer on a rimmed baking sheet for 20 minutes, then flip each piece and roast for an additional 10 to 15 minutes or until the beets are fork-tender and the edges are golden brown.

While the beets roast, melt the remaining 2 tablespoons bacon fat or coconut oil in a small skillet over medium heat. When the fat is hot, place the herbs in the pan and allow them to crisp for about 30 seconds, then serve them over the beets.

crumb-topped brussels sprouts

PREP TIME **15 MINS** • COOK TIME **40 MINS** • SERVINGS **4**

2 to 3 tablespoons coconut oil or bacon fat, melted

1 small head red or green cabbage, sliced into 1-inch-thick wedges

2 dozen Brussels sprouts, trimmed and cut in half lengthwise

1/2 teaspoon sea salt

1/2 teaspoon black pepper

FOR THE TOPPING

1/4 cup ground almonds or almond meal, store-bought* or homemade (page 213)

1/4 teaspoon onion powder

1/4 teaspoon granulated garlic

1/4 teaspoon ground cinnamon

1/2 teaspoon sea salt

1/2 teaspoon black pepper

INGREDIENT TIP
*Check out page 224 for a list of recommended brands. ●

NUTS

EGGS

NIGHTSHADES

FODMAPS

SEAFOOD

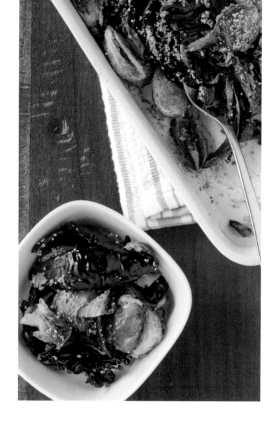

Preheat the oven to 375°F.

Pour a thin layer of the coconut oil or bacon fat in the bottom of a 9-inch-square baking dish, reserving the rest.

Arrange the cabbage and Brussels sprouts in the dish, sprinkle on the salt and pepper, then pour the remaining oil or fat over the top of the vegetables.

In a small bowl, combine the topping ingredients and set aside.

Bake the vegetables for 30 minutes, then remove from the oven and sprinkle the topping evenly over the veggies.

Bake for an additional 10 minutes or until the topping is lightly browned and the vegetables are tender.

herb almond "cheese" spread

PREP TIME **8 HRS + 10 MINS** • YIELD **2 CUPS**

1 cup raw almonds

2 1/4 cups water, divided

5 tablespoons extra-virgin olive oil

1/4 cup fresh lemon juice (2 lemons)

1 clove garlic, minced or grated

2 tablespoons minced fresh chives

sea salt and black pepper to taste

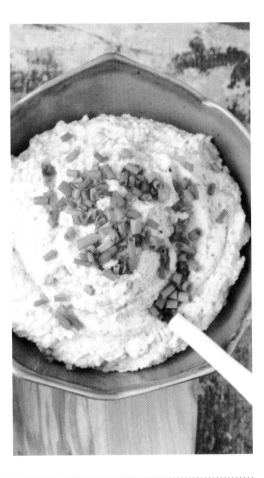

Place the almonds and 2 cups of the water in a glass or other nonporous container and let them soak, covered, in a dark place, overnight or for 8 hours.

Drain and rinse the almonds, then place them in a food processor along with the remaining 1/4 cup water and the rest of the ingredients. Process until smooth and creamy, stopping occasionally to scrape down the sides of the processor, about 5 minutes total.

If you'd like a lighter texture, add another tablespoon of warm water at a time until you achieve the desired consistency.

herb crackers

PREP TIME **30 MINS** • COOK TIME **10-15 MINS** • SERVINGS **4**

1 cup fine almond meal, store-bought* or homemade (page 213)

1/2 teaspoon sea salt

1/2 teaspoon onion powder

1/2 teaspoon granulated garlic

1 tablespoon chopped fresh herbs of your choice (see Chef Note)

black pepper to taste

1 egg, beaten

NUTS

EGGS

NIGHTSHADES

FODMAPS

SEAFOOD

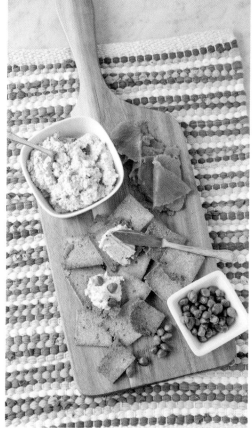

INGREDIENT TIP
*Check out page 224 for a list of recommended brands.

CHEF NOTE
Fresh chives and rosemary are good choices for these crackers. ●

Preheat the oven to 350°F.

In a mixing bowl, use a fork to combine the almond meal, salt, onion powder, granulated garlic, herbs, and pepper. Add the egg to the dry ingredients and combine with the fork until it forms a crumbly texture. Gather the dough into a ball, wrap it in a sheet of plastic wrap, and refrigerate for 20 to 30 minutes.

Remove the dough from the refrigerator, place it between 2 sheets of parchment paper, and roll it out gently with a rolling pin.

Use a knife or cookie cutter to make cracker shapes of your choice. Place the shapes on a baking sheet and bake for 10 to 15 minutes or until golden brown.

Allow the crackers to cool before serving with your favorite toppings.

simple beef jerky

PREP TIME **45 MINS** • DEHYDRATING TIME **3-5 HRS** • SERVINGS **VARIES**

FOR THE MARINADE

1/3 cup coconut aminos

1 teaspoon granulated garlic

1 teaspoon onion powder

1/2 teaspoon sea salt

1/4 teaspoon black pepper, or more to taste

1 pound lean beef (London broil or a roast with the fat trimmed works well), chicken, or turkey

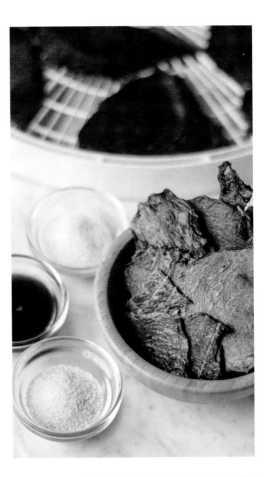

In a large bowl, whisk together the marinade ingredients. Taste it and adjust the seasonings as desired; it should taste stronger than you want the finished jerky to taste.

Cutting against the grain of the meat, slice the meat thinly into approximately 1/8-inch slices using a very sharp knife or a meat slicer.

Place the sliced meat in the marinade and allow it to sit at room temperature or in the refrigerator for up to 1 hour.

Arrange the meat on the trays of a food dehydrator and heat at 135°F to 145°F until the meat reaches the desired dryness. This should take approximately 3 to 5 hours.

To make jerky in the oven, set it to 200°F and bake for 2 to 4 hours until the jerky reaches desired level of dryness.

basic 4 guacamole

PREP TIME **10 MINS** • SERVINGS **8**

4 avocados

juice of 2 limes

1 medium shallot, minced

1/4 cup chopped fresh
  cilantro leaves

sea salt and black pepper to
  taste

1/2 jalapeño pepper,
  minced (optional; omit for
  nightshade free)

NUTS

EGGS

NIGHTSHADES

FODMAPS

SEAFOOD

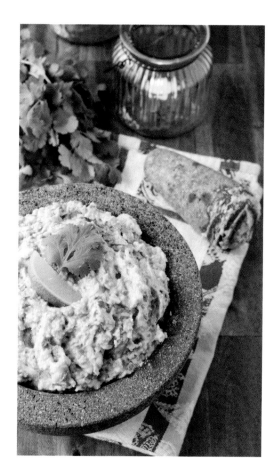

Slice each avocado in half lengthwise around the pit, remove the pit, then scoop the flesh into a mixing bowl. Mash the avocado with a fork.

Stir in the lime juice. Add the shallot, cilantro, salt, and pepper and stir until well combined. If you like spicy guacamole, add the jalapeño and stir to combine.

Serve chilled or at room temperature.

tomato & green onion faux-caccia

PREP TIME **15** • COOK TIME **50 MINS** • SERVINGS **8**

NUTS

EGGS

NIGHTSHADES

FODMAPS

SEAFOOD

6 eggs

1/2 teaspoon apple cider vinegar

1/2 cup unsalted butter, ghee, duck fat, or coconut oil, softened

1/2 cup coconut flour

1/4 teaspoon baking soda

1/2 teaspoon sea salt

1 tablespoon minced fresh basil leaves

1 tablespoon minced fresh rosemary

1 tablespoon dried oregano

2 to 3 cloves garlic, minced or grated

FOR THE SAUCE

1/4 cup tomato paste

1/4 cup water

1 to 2 cloves garlic, minced or grated

sea salt and black pepper to taste

2 tablespoons sliced green onion (scallion)

Preheat the oven to 350°F. Line a baking sheet with parchment paper.

In a large mixing bowl, whisk together the eggs, vinegar, and softened butter, ghee, duck fat, or coconut oil. Sift in the coconut flour, baking soda, and salt and whisk together until well combined.

Stir in the herbs and garlic, then spread the mixture over the prepared baking sheet.

Bake for 30 minutes or until the edges of the bread are golden brown.

While the bread bakes, make the sauce: In a small saucepan over medium-low heat, bring the tomato paste, water, garlic, salt, and pepper to a simmer and cook for approximately 10 minutes.

When the bread is done, spread the tomato sauce over the top in a thin, even layer, then sprinkle with the green onion.

Place back in the oven and bake for an additional 10 minutes.

KITCHEN TIP
The parchment paper is critical, as coconut flour has a very strong tendency to stick even to well-greased nonstick pans due to its high fiber content.

NIGHTSHADE FREE?
Omit the sauce.

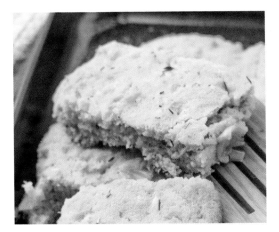

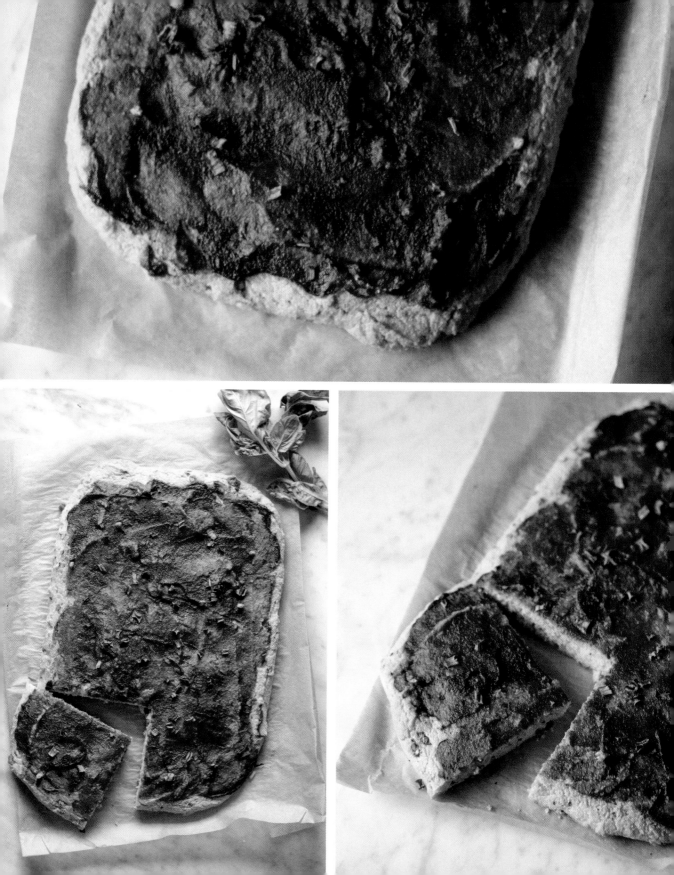

savory herb drop biscuits

PREP TIME **15 MINS** • COOK TIME **25 MINS** • SERVINGS **6**

• YIELD **6 MUFFINS OR 12 BISCUITS**

6 eggs

1/2 cup coconut oil or unsalted butter, melted but not hot

1/2 teaspoon apple cider vinegar

1/2 cup coconut flour

1/2 teaspoon baking soda

1/2 teaspoon sea salt

1 tablespoon fresh rosemary or sage leaves, chopped

Preheat the oven to 350°F.

In a mixing bowl, whisk together the eggs, coconut oil or butter, and vinegar until well combined.

Sift in the coconut flour, baking soda, and salt and stir to combine. Add the herbs and give it a quick stir.

Line a baking sheet with parchment paper and, using a large spoon, dollop the mixture onto the sheet in 12 small portions. Bake for 20 to 25 minutes or until golden brown.

To make as muffins: Line 6 cups of a muffin tin with parchment paper muffin cup liners and fill the cups evenly. Bake for approximately 25 minutes or until the muffins are set and the edges begin to become golden brown.

KITCHEN TIP
Don't skip the parchment! The parchment paper liners are critical, as coconut flour has a very strong tendency to stick even to well-greased nonstick muffin pans due to its high fiber content. If you can't find them, make this recipe as biscuits using a standard roll of parchment paper. ●

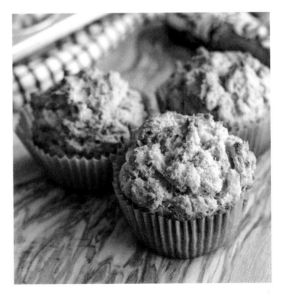

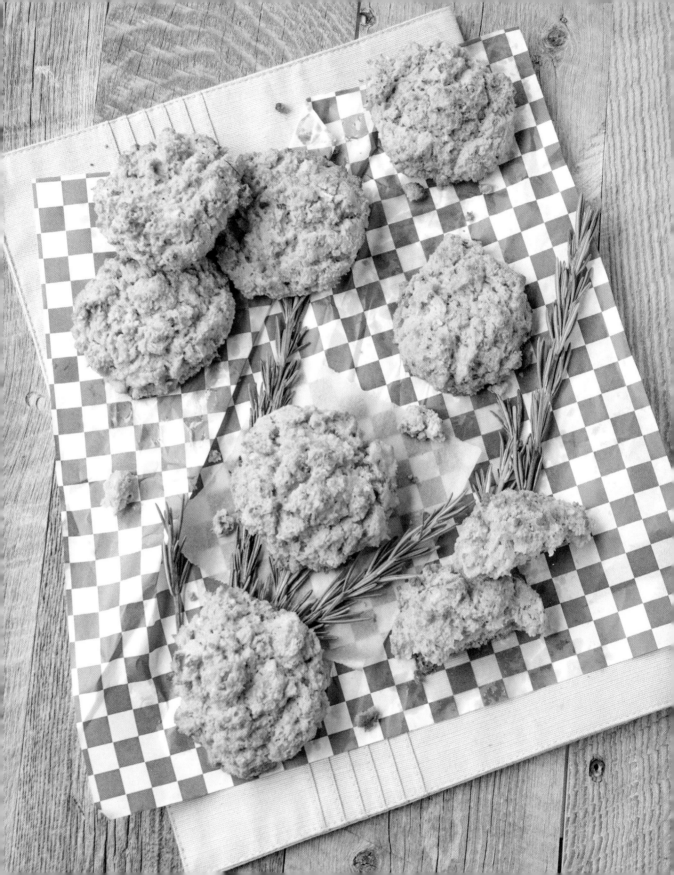

baked kale chips

PREP TIME **10 MINS** • COOK TIME **15-20 MINS** • SERVINGS **4**

1 large bunch curly kale

2 tablespoons coconut oil

1 to 2 cloves garlic, minced or grated

1 teaspoon onion powder

1/2 teaspoon paprika (optional)

3 tablespoons brewer's yeast* (optional)

2 tablespoons almond meal (use 4 to 5 tablespoons if omitting brewer's yeast), store-bought* or homemade (page 213)

sea salt and black pepper to taste

1/2 teaspoon granulated garlic

INGREDIENT TIP
*Check out page 224 for a list of recommended brands of almond meal. For brewer's yeast, I recommend Lewis Labs brand.

KITCHEN TIP
Baking kale on glass or ceramic cookware tends to yield a more "wet" result, and the chips don't bake up as easily. This is why I recommend metal baking sheets.

NIGHTSHADE FREE?
Omit the paprika. ●

Preheat the oven to 350°F.

Holding the stem of each kale leaf with one hand, use your other hand to rip both sides of the leaf from the stem. Discard the stems. Rinse the kale, then thoroughly pat it dry with paper towels and/or spread it out and allow it to dry for several hours.

In a small mixing bowl, combine the coconut oil, garlic, onion powder, paprika (if using), brewer's yeast (if using), almond meal, salt, and pepper.

In a large mixing bowl, toss half of the well-dried kale with half of the spice mixture, massaging it into the leaves, then arrange the kale in a single layer on a metal baking sheet (without a nonstick surface). Repeat with the second half of the kale and spice blend and spread evenly onto a second baking sheet. Sprinkle the kale with a little extra salt and the granulated garlic.

Bake for 15 to 20 minutes or until the kale becomes crispy but not browned. If after 20 minutes of baking the kale still seems a bit soggy (which often happens if the kale was not completely dry before baking), simply turn off the oven and leave the kale in the oven while it cools down for an additional 20 minutes. This will give the kale more time to dry out.

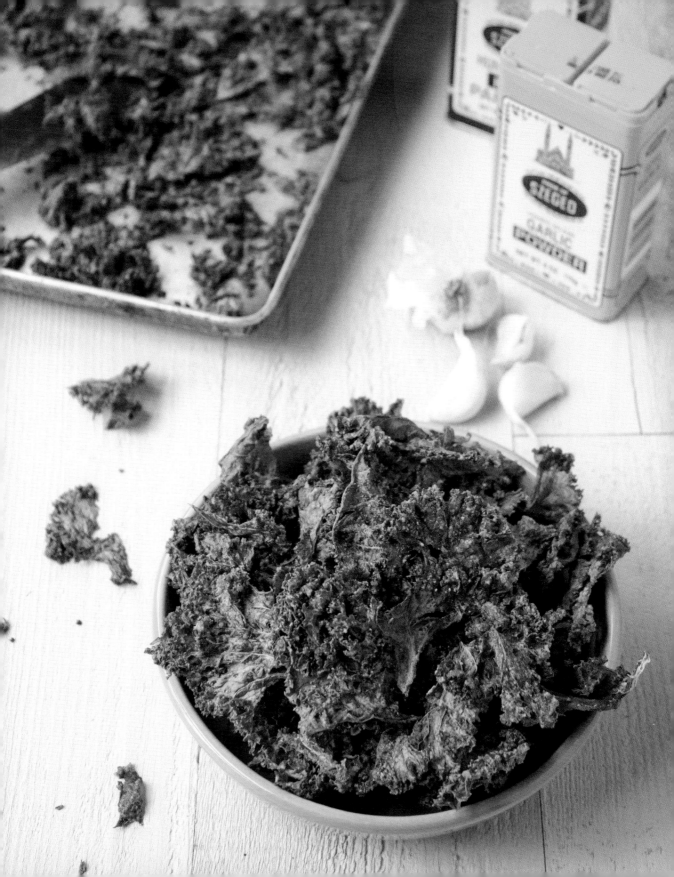

cinnilla nut mix

PREP TIME **5 MINS** · COOK TIME **25-30 MINS** · SERVINGS **4**

NUTS
EGGS
NIGHTSHADES
FODMAPS
SEAFOOD

1 egg white

1 tablespoon coconut oil, melted

1/4 teaspoon pure vanilla extract

1 teaspoon ground cinnamon

2 pinches of sea salt

1/4 cup almonds

1/4 cup macadamia nuts

1/2 cup walnuts

2 tablespoons almond meal, store-bought* or homemade (page 213)

Preheat the oven to 275°F.

In a mixing bowl, whisk together the egg white, coconut oil, vanilla, cinnamon, and salt. Add the nuts (you may substitute others of your choice) and almond meal, and toss to evenly coat.

Spread evenly on a rimmed baking sheet and bake for 25 to 30 minutes or until toasted.

INGREDIENT TIP
*Check out page 224 for a list of recommended brands. ●

NUTS
EGGS
NIGHTSHADES
FODMAPS
SEAFOOD

spicy thai nut mix

PREP TIME **5 MINS** · COOK TIME **25-30 MINS** · SERVINGS **4**

1 tablespoon coconut aminos*

1 tablespoon coconut oil, melted

2 to 4 drops fish sauce*

zest and juice of 1 lime

1/4 teaspoon cayenne pepper

1/8 teaspoon minced fresh ginger, or more to taste

1/4 cup almonds

1/4 cup pepitas (pumpkin seeds)

1/2 cup walnuts

1 teaspoon sesame seeds

Preheat the oven to 275°F.

In a mixing bowl, whisk together the coconut aminos, coconut oil, fish sauce, lime zest, lime juice, cayenne pepper, and ginger. Add the nuts and seeds (you may substitute others of your choice), and toss to evenly coat.

Spread evenly on a baking sheet and bake for 25 to 30 minutes or until toasted.

INGREDIENT TIP
*Check out page 224 for a list of recommended brands. ●

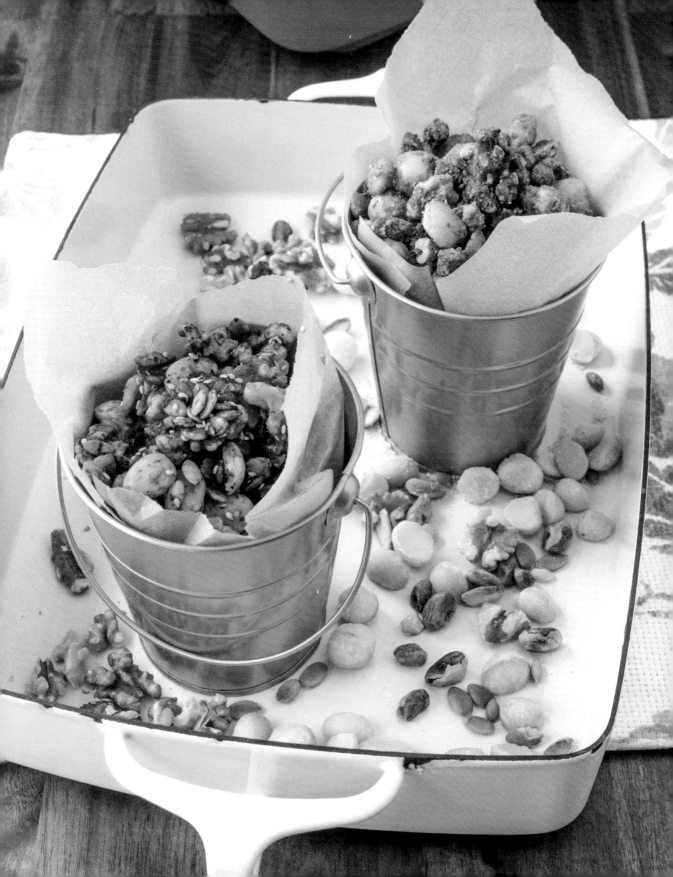

tart & creamy applesauce

PREP TIME **15 MINS** • COOK TIME **20 MINS** • SERVINGS **8**

NUTS

EGGS

NIGHTSHADES

FODMAPS

SEAFOOD

8 green apples, peeled and chopped into 1/2-inch pieces

zest and juice of 2 lemons

1/2 cup unsalted butter

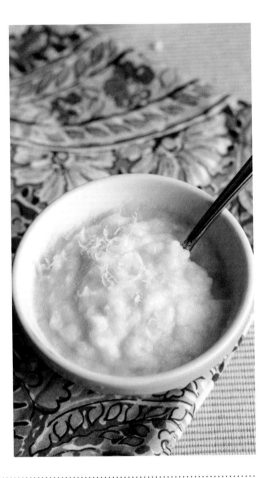

KITCHEN TIP

Use coconut oil if you can't tolerate butter. However, the applesauce may harden in the refrigerator and will need to come to room temperature again before you can enjoy it. ●

In an enameled cast-iron or stainless-steel pot, combine the apples, lemon zest, lemon juice, and butter. Simmer over medium heat until the fruit is soft, approximately 15 to 20 minutes.

Mash or purée the apples to whatever texture you like, or leave it chunky.

Serve warm or at room temperature. It will solidify a bit as it cools.

not-sweet cinnamon cookies

PREP TIME **10 MINS** • COOK TIME **15 MINS** • SERVINGS **4** • YIELD **8 COOKIES**

1/4 cup mashed green-tipped banana (approximately 1 small)

2 eggs

2 teaspoons coconut oil or unsalted butter, melted

1/2 teaspoon pure vanilla extract

1 tablespoon coconut flour

1 teaspoon ground cinnamon

1 cup unsweetened shredded coconut

pinch of sea salt

NUTS

EGGS

NIGHTSHADES

FODMAPS

SEAFOOD

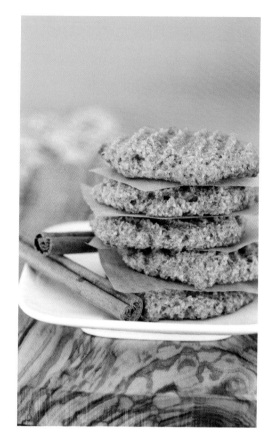

Preheat the oven to 350°F. Line a baking sheet with parchment paper.

In a medium-sized mixing bowl, whisk together the banana, eggs, coconut oil or butter, and vanilla.

Sift the coconut flour and cinnamon over the egg mixture and stir to combine. Mix in the shredded coconut and salt.

Spoon the cookies onto the prepared baking sheet in 8 evenly sized dollops, then flatten with a fork.

Bake until golden brown, about 15 minutes.

vanilla bean coconut freezer pops

PREP TIME **5 MINS** • SERVINGS **VARIES**

NUTS

EGGS

NIGHTSHADES

FODMAPS

SEAFOOD

1 (14.5-ounce) can full-fat coconut milk*

water to fill ice pop molds (see Kitchen Tip to determine quantity)

1 vanilla bean pod

1 teaspoon pure vanilla extract

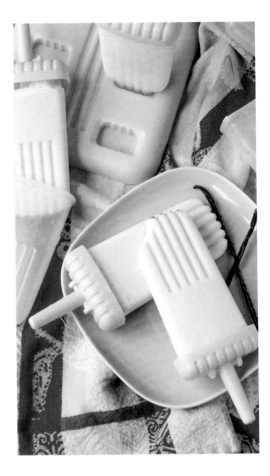

INGREDIENT TIP

*Check out page 224 for a list of recommended brands.

SPECIAL EQUIPMENT

Ice pop molds are pretty easy to find in home stores and are also available online at shops like Amazon.com and Target.com. Visit The 21-Day Sugar Detox shop online to find more useful gadgets, tools, and helpful items: balancedbites.com/21DSD.

KITCHEN TIP

To calculate how much water you'll need to add, fill an ice pop mold to capacity, then measure the liquid in a measuring cup. Multiply that amount by the number of pops you have. Since you have only 14.5 ounces of coconut milk for all the pops, you can add water to make up the difference. For example, if you have 6 pop holders and each one holds 3 ounces of liquid, you will need 18 ounces of liquid. In this case, you will want to add 3.5 ounces of water to the 14.5 ounces of coconut milk to give you a total of 18 ounces. ●

Pour the coconut milk into a mixing bowl (preferably one with an easy-pour spout) or into a blender. Add the amount of water needed to top off your ice pop molds (see the Kitchen Tip to determine the amount).

Slice the vanilla bean pod in half lengthwise, then scrape the back of your knife down the inside of the pod to remove the seeds.

Place the vanilla bean seeds in the bowl or blender with the coconut milk and water, then add the vanilla extract and either whisk together or blend.

Pour evenly into the molds and freeze overnight. To remove the pops, run the containers under warm water until the sides release.

banana coconut ice cream

PREP TIME **6 HRS + 10 MINS** • SERVINGS **4**

4 green-tipped bananas

2 tablespoons coconut butter*

2 teaspoons pure vanilla extract

seeds from 1 vanilla bean pod

OPTIONAL GARNISHES

2 tablespoons 100% dark chocolate shavings (pictured)

2 tablespoons cacao nibs

2 tablespoons unsweetened shredded coconut

INGREDIENT TIP
*Check out page 224 for a list of recommended brands. ●

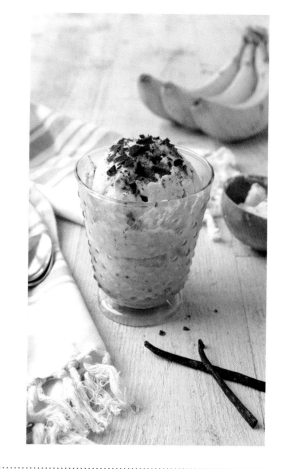

NOT-SWEET TREATS

NUTS

EGGS

NIGHTSHADES

FODMAPS

SEAFOOD

Peel the green bananas and chop them into 1-inch pieces, then freeze them for at least 6 hours or overnight.

In a small bowl, stir together the coconut butter, vanilla extract, and vanilla bean seeds.

Place the frozen bananas and the coconut butter mixture in a food processor and process for 1 to 2 minutes or until the mixture looks like minced pieces, stopping to scrape the sides of the container as needed.

Transfer the mixture to a mixing bowl and stir with a large spoon. The mixture should begin to meld and develop more of a creamy texture. Scoop into 4 serving dishes and top with the optional garnishes, if using.

NUTS

EGGS

NIGHTSHADES

FODMAPS

SEAFOOD

bittersweet hot cocoa

PREP TIME **5 MINS** · COOK TIME **5 MINS** · SERVINGS **4**

1 1/2 cups full-fat coconut milk*

1 1/2 cups water

1/2 cup plus 1 tablespoon unsweetened cocoa powder*

1/2 teaspoon pure vanilla extract

seeds from 1 vanilla pod (optional)

a few pinches of ground cinnamon (optional)

INGREDIENT TIP
*Check out page 224 for a list of recommended brands. ●

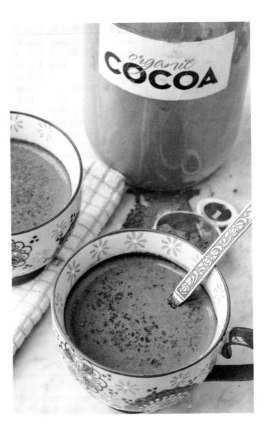

In a saucepan, whisk together all the ingredients and bring to a simmer over medium heat. Serve hot.

You may also want to chill this cocoa and use it as a base for a smoothie or not-sweet chocolate freezer pops.

apple cinnamon donuts

PREP TIME **20 MINS** • COOK TIME **30 MINS** • SERVINGS **6**
• YIELD **6 REGULAR OR 12 MINI DONUTS**

2 tablespoons melted
unsalted butter or ghee

3 tablespoons coconut oil,
divided

1 green apple, peeled and
diced

3 eggs

1/2 teaspoon pure vanilla
extract

5 tablespoons full-fat coconut
milk*

1/2 teaspoon apple cider
vinegar

1/4 cup coconut flour,* sifted

1/3 cup almond flour*

1/2 teaspoon baking soda

1 teaspoon ground cinnamon

2 pinches of sea salt

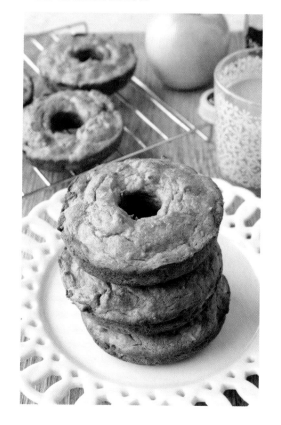

NUTS

EGGS

NIGHTSHADES

FODMAPS

SEAFOOD

Preheat the oven to 350°F. Brush a 6-cavity donut pan or 12-cavity mini-donut pan with the butter or ghee.

In a skillet over medium heat, melt 1 tablespoon of the coconut oil. Sauté the apple until soft, approximately 8 to 10 minutes. Place the cooked apple in the refrigerator to chill for at least 5 minutes.

In a mixing bowl, vigorously whisk the eggs, vanilla, the remaining 2 tablespoons coconut oil, coconut milk, and vinegar for about 20 seconds until combined. Add the coconut flour, almond flour, baking soda, cinnamon, cooked apples, and salt to the egg mixture and whisk vigorously until smooth.

Pour the batter into the prepared donut pan, filling each cavity about two-thirds of the way full, as the donuts will puff up while baking.

Bake for 20 minutes or until the donuts are puffed-up and golden brown.

Note: Each regular-sized donut includes 1/6 of a green apple; each mini donut, 1/12 of an apple. Factor this into your total intake of allowed fruit for the day.

INGREDIENT TIP
*Check out page 224 for a list of recommended brands.

SPECIAL EQUIPMENT
You can find donut pans at most major home stores as well as online. Visit balancedbites.com/21DSD for recommended brands. ●

grain-free banola

PREP TIME **10 MINS** • COOK TIME **30-35 MINS** • SERVINGS **8**

NUTS

EGGS

NIGHTSHADES

FODMAPS

SEAFOOD

2 cups whole or halved nuts of choice (walnuts, pecans, macadamias, almonds)

1 cup slivered or sliced almonds

1/2 cup seeds of choice (pumpkin, sunflower, sesame)

1/2 cup almond or other nut meal

2 green-tipped bananas (to yield about 1 cup when puréed)

1 egg

2 teaspoons pure vanilla extract

2 teaspoons cinnamon

1/2 teaspoon nutmeg (optional)

1/4 teaspoon sea salt

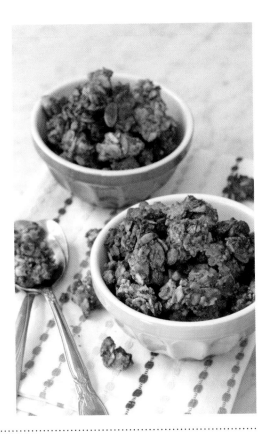

Preheat the oven to 350°F.

In a food processor, pulse the whole or halved nuts until they're partially ground and partially still in small chunks. Pour the nuts into a large mixing bowl, then stir in the slivered almonds, seeds, and almond meal.

Place the bananas, egg, vanilla, cinnamon, nutmeg (if using), and sea salt into the food processor and process for 20 seconds or until all the ingredients are puréed. Pour the banana mixture into the nut mixture and stir until the nuts are well coated.

Pour the nut mixture onto a parchment paper–lined baking sheet.

Bake in the oven for about 30 to 35 minutes, checking every 10 minutes and turning the chunks of granola with a large spoon to break up the very large pieces. This allows it to dry out and lightly brown on all sides. Remove from the oven and let cool, uncovered, or turn off the oven and allow it to continue to dehydrate as the oven cools. Store in the refrigerator for up to a week. Enjoy it plain as a snack, or with coconut or almond milk as a cereal.

nutty baked apples

PREP TIME **10 MINS** • COOK TIME **30 MINS** • SERVINGS **4**

4 green apples

1 cup coarsely ground nuts of your choice (use one or more of the following: almonds, walnuts, pecans, shelled pistachios, macadamia nuts)

1 teaspoon ground cinnamon

a few pinches of sea salt

1/4 cup plus 2 tablespoons unsalted butter, ghee, or coconut oil, melted

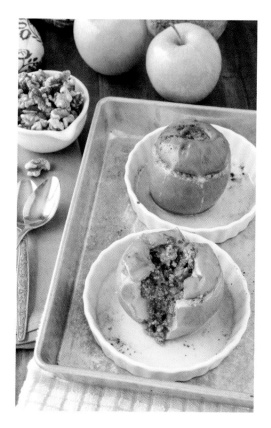

NUTS

EGGS

NIGHTSHADES

FODMAPS

SEAFOOD

Preheat the oven to 350°F.

Slice off roughly the top 1/4-inch of each apple. Core the apples, leaving about 3/4-inch of the bottom of the apple intact. Place the apples in a 9 by 9-inch baking dish.

In a small mixing bowl, combine the ground nuts, cinnamon, salt, and butter, ghee, or coconut oil and mix until the nuts are evenly coated. Stuff each of the apples with the nut mixture, then bake until the skins of the apples just break open and the apples appear completely soft and slightly golden brown, approximately 30 minutes.

NUTS

EGGS

NIGHTSHADES

FODMAPS

SEAFOOD

lemon vanilla meltaways

PREP TIME **10 MINS** • SERVINGS **4** • YIELD **12 PIECES**

1/2 cup coconut butter*, softened

1/2 cup coconut oil, softened

seeds from 1/2 vanilla bean pod

zest and juice of 1 lemon

INGREDIENT TIP
*Check out page 224 for a list of recommended brands. ●

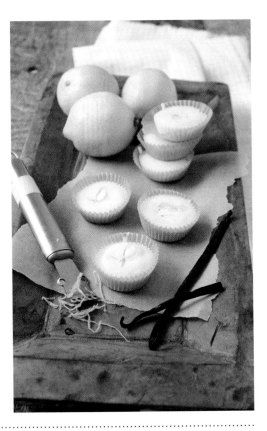

Line 12 cups of a mini-muffin tin with mini parchment paper liners.

In a mixing bowl (preferably one with a spout), whisk together the coconut butter, coconut oil, vanilla bean seeds, lemon zest, and lemon juice until well combined.

Pour the mixture into the prepared muffin tin and chill for 20 to 30 minutes or until completely solid. Serve 3 pieces per person.

moo-less chocolate mousse

PREP TIME **10 MINS** • SERVINGS **2**

1 avocado

1 medium-large green-tipped banana

1/4 cup full-fat coconut, almond, or other milk

1/4 cup unsweetened cocoa powder* or unsweetened carob powder

1/4 teaspoon pure vanilla extract

OPTIONAL FLAVORINGS

pinch of sea salt

dash of ground cinnamon

OPTIONAL GARNISHES

1 tablespoon 100% dark chocolate shavings

1 tablespoon cacao nibs

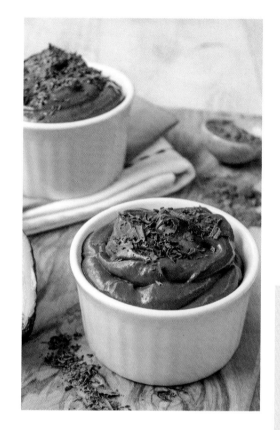

NUTS

EGGS

NIGHTSHADES

FODMAPS

SEAFOOD

INGREDIENT TIP
*Check out page 224 for a list of recommended brands.

KITCHEN TIP
If you have a handheld immersion blender, you may use that or the mini-food processor attachment that often comes with it. If you would like to use a large food processor, I recommend doubling the recipe. You could also whisk this mousse by hand or with beaters. ●

Halve the avocado and remove the pit. Scoop out the flesh into a small food processor along with the banana, milk, cocoa or carob powder, and vanilla extract.

Add the salt and/or cinnamon, if using, and blend until completely smooth, scraping down the sides once or twice.

Serve in individual bowls and garnish as desired.

granny smith apple crumble

PREP TIME **15 MINS** • COOK TIME **45-50 MINS** • SERVINGS **4**

NUTS

EGGS

NIGHTSHADES

FODMAPS

SEAFOOD

FOR THE FILLING

4 green apples, peeled and
   thinly sliced

juice of 1/2 lemon

1 teaspoon ground
   cinnamon

FOR THE TOPPING

1 1/4 cups almond meal or
   other nut meal of your
   choice, store-bought* or
   homemade (page 213)

1/4 cup unsalted butter or
   coconut oil, softened

1 teaspoon ground
   cinnamon

pinch of sea salt

1 tablespoon unsalted
   butter or coconut oil,
   melted, for the pan

Preheat the oven to 350°F.

Make the filling: In a mixing bowl, toss the apples with the lemon juice and cinnamon.

Make the topping: In a separate bowl, mix together the almond meal, butter or coconut oil, cinnamon, and salt until completely incorporated.

Brush the bottom and sides of a 9 by 9-inch or similar-sized baking dish with the melted butter or coconut oil.

Place the apples in the baking dish and cover evenly with the topping.

Bake for 20 minutes covered with foil, then for an additional 25 to 30 minutes uncovered, until the apples are soft and the topping begins to brown on the edges.

INGREDIENT TIP

*Check out page 224 for a list of recommended brands.

CHEF NOTE

If you're like me, you'll find yourself returning to this recipe even after you've completed The 21DSD. It's the perfect super-simple after-dinner treat that's not too sweet. ●

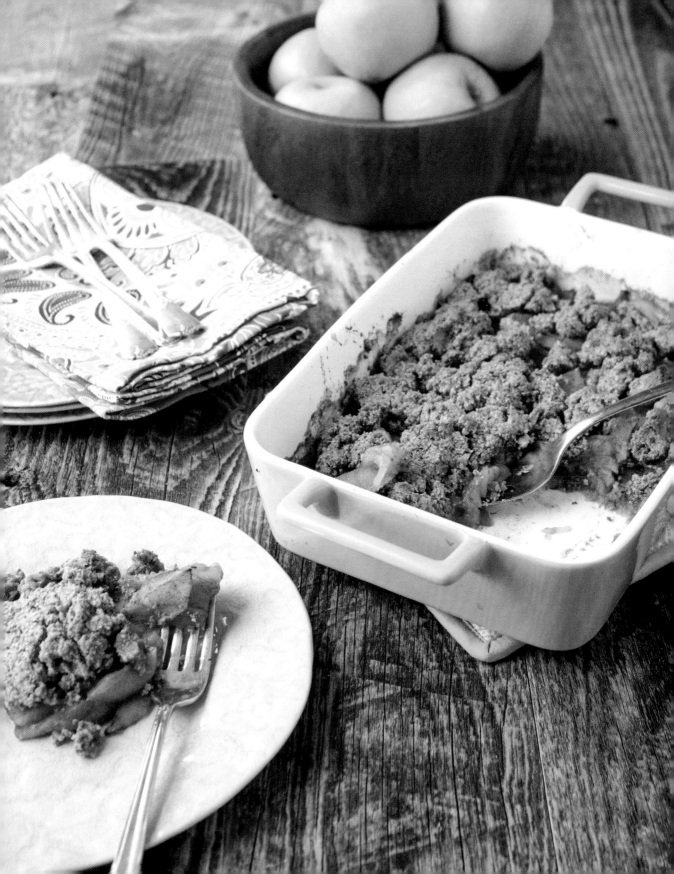

NUTS

EGGS

NIGHTSHADES

FODMAPS

SEAFOOD

almond butter cups

PREP TIME **15 MINS** • SERVINGS **6** • YIELD **12 PIECES**

FOR THE SHELLS

1/4 cup coconut oil, melted

1/4 cup coconut butter,* softened

1/2 cup unsweetened cocoa powder*

1/2 teaspoon pure vanilla extract

pinch of sea salt

pinch of ground cinnamon

FOR THE FILLING

3 tablespoons almond butter* or other nut butter

1 tablespoon coconut oil

pinch of sea salt

INGREDIENT TIP
*Check out page 224 for a list of recommended brands. ●

Line 12 cups of a mini-muffin tin with mini parchment paper liners.

Make the shells: In a medium-sized mixing bowl, whisk together all the ingredients for the shells. Spoon a 1/8-inch layer (approximately 1 teaspoon) of the shell mixture into the bottom of each of the prepared cups. Place the tin in the refrigerator or freezer to set.

While the first layer of the shells is setting up, make the filling: Combine all the ingredients for the filling in a small mixing bowl.

Place the filling mixture into a 1-quart plastic bag or a pastry bag. Snip off a tiny corner of the bag with scissors.

Remove the shells from the refrigerator or freezer, and begin to pipe a small amount (about 1/2 teaspoon) of the filling into the center of each one, leaving some of the edge visible.

Once all the shells have been filled, cover the filling with an even layer of the remaining shell mixture.

Place the muffin tin back in the refrigerator or freezer to set, and serve cold or at room temperature.

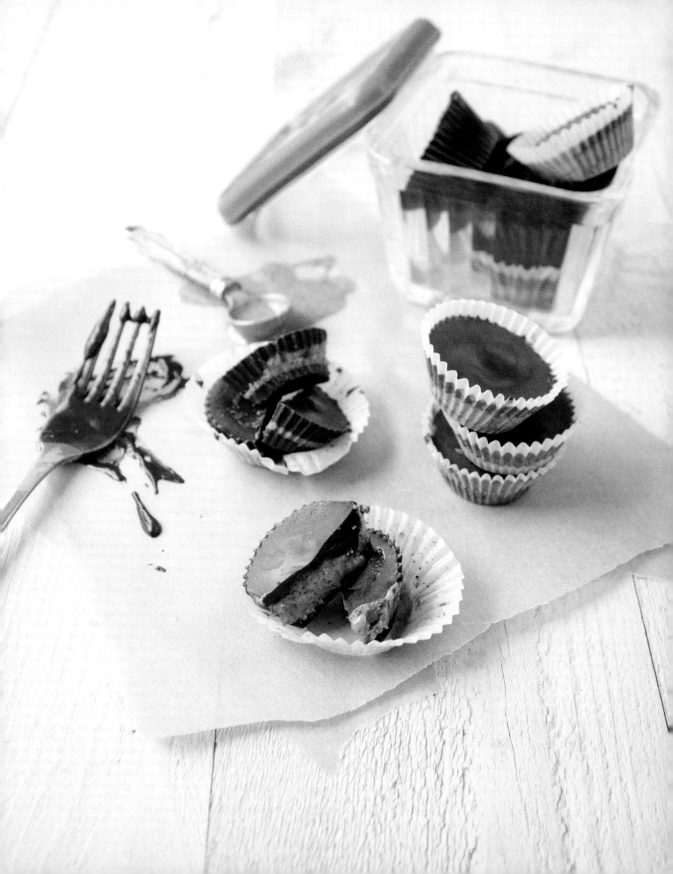

spice blends

Use these blends as they appear in recipes throughout the book—or use them anytime!

SMOKY SPICE BLEND
1 tablespoon chipotle powder
1 tablespoon smoked paprika
1 tablespoon onion powder
1/2 tablespoon cinnamon
1 tablespoon sea salt
1/2 tablespoon black pepper

PREP TIME **5 MINS** • YIELD **5 TABLESPOONS**

Combine all the spices in a bowl, and store them in a small container.

ITALIAN SAUSAGE SPICE BLEND
1 teaspoon sea salt
1 tablespoon fennel seeds, ground
1 tablespoon ground sage
1 tablespoon granulated garlic
1 tablespoon onion powder
1/4 teaspoon white pepper (or 1 teaspoon black pepper)
2 teaspoons dried parsley (optional)

PREP TIME **5 MINS** • YIELD **5 TABLESPOONS**

Combine all the spices in a bowl, and store them in a small container.

Use 2 tablespoons per pound of meat to make sausage.

CHORIZO SPICE BLEND
2 tablespoons chipotle powder
1 tablespoon smoked paprika
1 tablespoon onion powder
1 tablespoon granulated garlic
1/2 tablespoon sea salt
1 teaspoon black pepper

PREP TIME **5 MINS** • YIELD **6 TABLESPOONS**

Combine all the spices in a bowl, and store them in a small container.

Use 2 tablespoons of Chorizo spice blend, plus 1 tablespoon of apple cider vinegar per pound of meat.

SWEET & SAVORY SPICE BLEND
1 tablespoon granulated garlic
1 tablespoon onion powder
1 tablespoon cinnamon
1 tablespoon paprika
1 teaspoon cumin
1 tablespoon black pepper
2 teaspoons sea salt

PREP TIME **5 MINS** • YIELD **6 TABLESPOONS**

Combine all the spices in a bowl, and store them in a small container.

NIGHTSHADE FREE?
Omit the following from your blends: paprika, chili powder, chipotle powder, and red pepper flakes.

FODMAP FREE?
Eliminate the onion powder and granulated garlic. ●

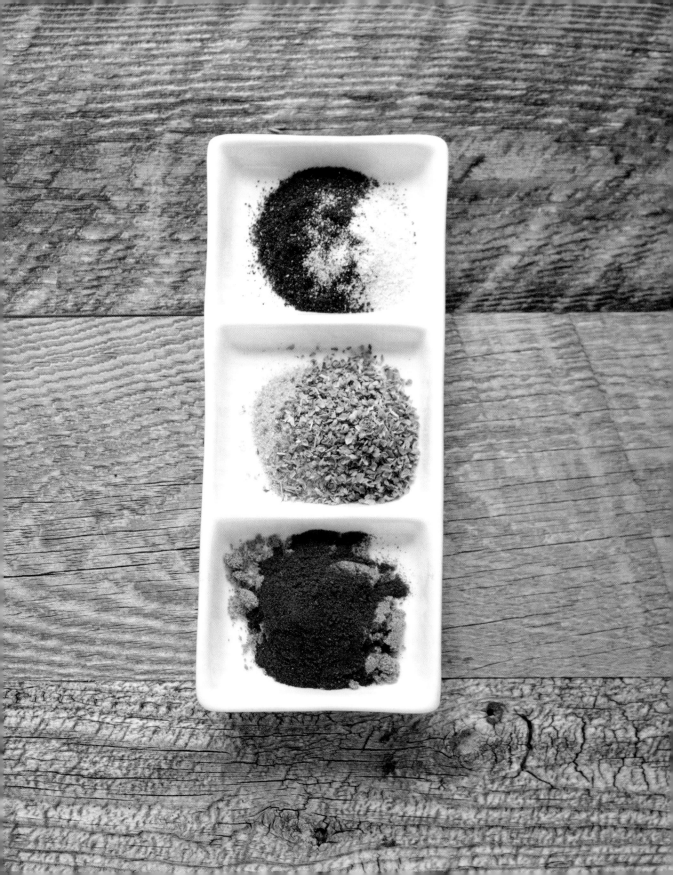

clarified butter & ghee

PREP TIME **5 MINS** • COOK TIME **25-30 MINS (CLARIFIED BUTTER), 35-45 MINS (GHEE)** •
YIELD **25-30 OUNCES**

2 pounds unsalted butter
from pastured cows
(brands I like include
Kerrygold, SMJÖR, Organic
Pastures, and Organic
Valley Pasture Butter)

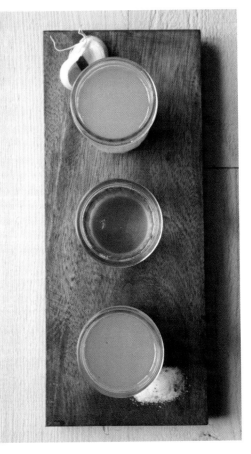

**KEEP IT COOL,
OR DON'T**
Clarified butter and
ghee, when properly
prepared, are shelf
stable. If you didn't
remove all the
milk solids or the
temperature in your
home becomes very
warm, it may go off
sooner than you like.
You can refrigerate
these to make them
last longer. ●

To make clarified butter: Place
the butter in a medium-sized,
heavyweight saucepan, and melt it
slowly over low heat. As the butter
comes to a simmer, the milk solids
will float to the top and become
foamy while the separated oil will
become very clear. Skim off the milk
solids, and remove the butter from
the heat. Pour it through cheesecloth
to strain out any remaining milk
solids, and store the strained liquid in
a glass jar.

To make ghee: Follow the
instructions for making clarified
butter, but allow the milk solids to
continue to cook slowly until they
become browned and begin to sink
to the bottom of the pan. When there
are no longer any solids waiting to
brown and sink to the bottom of
the oil, the ghee is finished. Pour it
through cheesecloth to strain out the
browned milk solids, and store the
strained liquid in a glass jar.

healthy homemade mayonnaise

PREP TIME 15 MINS • **YIELD 3/4 CUP**

2 egg yolks

1 tablespoon fresh lemon juice

1 teaspoon gluten-free Dijon mustard*

1/2 cup macadamia nut oil or other oil (page 61)

1/4 cup extra-virgin olive oil

NUTS

EGGS

NIGHTSHADES

FODMAPS

SEAFOOD

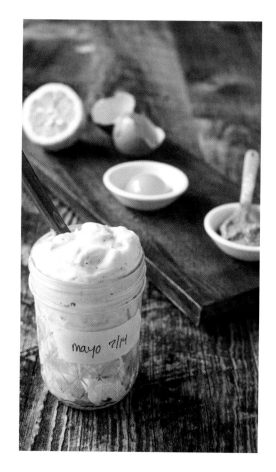

INGREDIENT TIP
*Check out page 224 for a list of recommended brands.

KITCHEN TIP
You can also make this recipe using a handheld immersion blender or a small blender. If using a regular-sized blender, double the recipe to make blending easier. Use the opening at the top of your blender to slowly drizzle in the oil. ●

In a medium-sized mixing bowl, whisk together the egg yolks, lemon juice, and mustard until blended and bright yellow, about 30 seconds. Begin adding 1/4 cup of the macadamia nut oil to the yolk mixture a few drops at a time, whisking constantly. Gradually add the remaining 1/4 cup macadamia nut oil and the olive oil in a slow, thin stream, whisking constantly, until the mayonnaise is thick and lighter in color.

Store in the refrigerator for up to a week.

bone broth

PREP TIME **5 MINS** • COOK TIME **8-24 HRS** • YIELD **ABOUT 2 1/2 QTS**

4 quarts filtered water

1 1/2 to 2 pounds bones (beef knuckle bones, marrow bones, meaty bones, chicken or turkey necks, chicken or turkey carcass bones, or any bones you have on hand)

2 tablespoons apple cider vinegar*

2 teaspoons sea salt

cloves from 1 whole head garlic, peeled and smashed (optional)

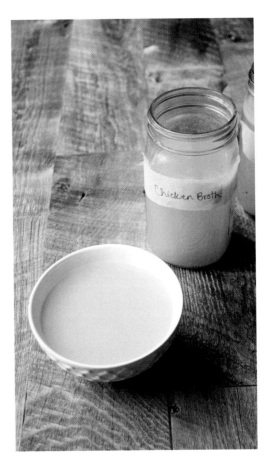

INGREDIENT TIP
*Check out page 224 for a list of recommended brands.

FODMAP FREE?
Omit the garlic. ●

Place all the ingredients in a 6-quart slow cooker. Turn the heat to high and bring the water to a boil. Then reduce the heat to low. Allow the broth to cook for a minimum of 8 hours and up to 24 hours. The longer it cooks, the better.

Turn off the slow cooker and allow the broth to cool to room temperature. Strain the broth through a fine-mesh strainer or a colander lined with cheesecloth. Store the broth in glass jars in the refrigerator for up to a week, or freeze for later use.

Before using the broth, chip away at the top and discard any fat that has solidified. You can drink the broth or use it as a base for soups, stews, or any recipe that calls for soup stock or broth.

almond milk & meal

PREP TIME **8 HRS + 10 MINS** · YIELD **2 CUPS**

2 cups raw almonds

7 cups water, divided

OPTIONAL FLAVORINGS

1/2 to 1 teaspoon pure vanilla extract (recommended)

1/2 teaspoon cinnamon

1/2 teaspoon unsweetened cocoa powder*

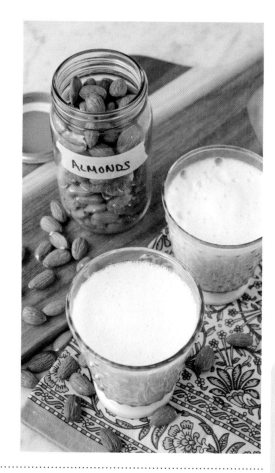

NUTS

EGGS

NIGHTSHADES

FODMAPS

SEAFOOD

INGREDIENT TIP
*Check out page 224 for a list of recommended brands.

SPECIAL EQUIPMENT
A nut milk bag is made of fine mesh cloth and is designed expressly for the purpose of making this type of milk. Visit balancedbites. com/21DSD for recommended brands.

KITCHEN TIP
This recipe works best in a powerful, high-speed blender like a Blendtec or Vitamix. ●

To make almond milk: Place the almonds and 4 cups of the water in a glass or other nonporous container and let them soak, covered, in a dark place, overnight or for 8 hours.

Strain and rinse the almonds in clean water.

Place the rinsed almonds in a blender with the remaining 3 cups water and blend on high for 2 minutes. Strain the liquid through a nut milk bag or layered cheesecloth over a bowl to catch the milk. Reserve the strained meal. If using optional flavorings, rinse out the blender, place the milk back in with the flavorings, and pulse to combine.

Store almond milk in the refrigerator for up to 5 days.

To make almond meal: Dehydrate the strained meal in a 170°F to 200°F oven for 3 to 4 hours or until completely dry. Pulse in a food processor to smooth out clumps, and store in the refrigerator to use when almond meal is called for in recipes.

sweetener-free ketchup

PREP TIME **10 MINS** • COOK TIME **4 HRS** • YIELD **16 OUNCES**

1 small onion, diced

2 green/granny smith apples, peeled and diced

2 cloves garlic, minced

1/2 teaspoon sea salt

1/4 teaspoon allspice

1/4 teaspoon cinnamon

2 pinches of cloves

1/4 teaspoon ginger powder

2 tablespoons apple cider vinegar

1/4 cup water

6 ounces tomato paste

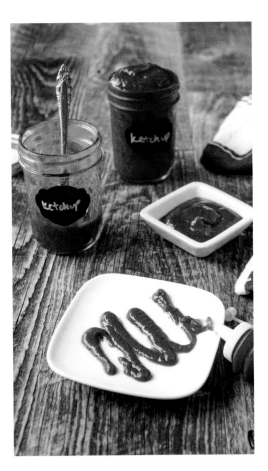

Place all the ingredients in a slow cooker and stir to combine. Set the slow cooker to low and cook for 4 hours.

Allow the mixture to cool slightly, then pour into a food processor or high-speed blender and blend until smooth.

Note: When blending or processing warm foods, do not overfill the container, as the heat will cause the contents to expand and they may splatter out.

Once blended, place the ketchup in glass containers and allow it to come to room temperature before refrigerating.

The ketchup should last for several weeks or more in the refrigerator. If you notice a change in color or smell or see any mold growth, toss it and make new batch.

simple marinara

PREP TIME **10 MINS** • COOK TIME **30 MINS** • SERVINGS **4**
• YIELD ABOUT **24 OUNCES**

2 tablespoons bacon fat,
lard, coconut oil, or other
cooking fat

1/2 cup diced yellow onion

sea salt and black pepper to
taste

2 to 3 cloves garlic, grated or
minced

28 ounces diced tomatoes

1 tablespoon chopped fresh
basil leaves

2 tablespoons extra-virgin
olive oil, to finish

NUTS

EGGS

NIGHTSHADES

FODMAPS

SEAFOOD

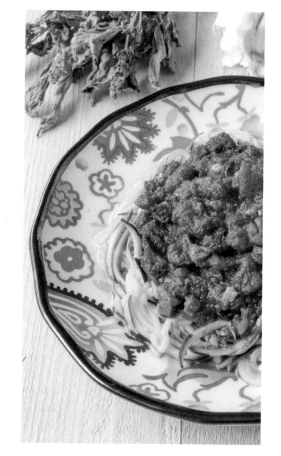

In a saucepan, melt the cooking fat over medium heat, and cook the onion until it is translucent, approximately 5 minutes. Season with salt and pepper.

Add the garlic and cook for an additional 30 seconds. Add the tomatoes, season with additional salt and pepper, and stir to combine. Reduce the heat to low and simmer for 15 to 20 minutes.

Add the basil and simmer for an additional 5 minutes.

Serve over zucchini noodles (pictured). Finish with a drizzle of extra-virgin olive oil for added flavor and richness.

For all sauces and dressings, combine all the ingredients in a small mixing bowl and whisk together vigorously. Store in a sealed glass jar in the refrigerator for up to 1 week.

avo-goddess sauce

PREP TIME **5 MINS** • SERVINGS **4** • YIELD **ABOUT 1/2 CUP**

NUTS
EGGS
NIGHTSHADES
FODMAPS
SEAFOOD

1/2 avocado
1/4 cup full-fat coconut
  milk*
juice of 1/2 lemon

1/2 clove garlic, minced or grated
1 to 2 teaspoons chopped fresh chives
sea salt and black pepper to taste

creamy ginger lime dressing

PREP TIME **5 MINS** • SERVINGS **4** • YIELD **ABOUT 1/2 CUP**

NUTS
EGGS
NIGHTSHADES
FODMAPS
SEAFOOD

1/2 to 1 teaspoon minced
  fresh ginger
zest and juice of 1/2 lime

1/4 cup full-fat coconut milk*
1/4 cup + 2 tablespoons macadamia nut oil

spicy sesame ginger dressing

PREP TIME **5 MINS** • SERVINGS **4** • YIELD **ABOUT 1/2 CUP**

NUTS
EGGS
NIGHTSHADES
FODMAPS
SEAFOOD

1/4 cup cold-pressed
  sesame oil
juice of 2 limes

1/2 to 1 teaspoon minced fresh ginger
pinch of red chili flakes, or to taste
sea salt and black pepper to taste

avo-ziki sauce

PREP TIME **5 MINS** • SERVINGS **4** • YIELD **ABOUT 1/2 CUP**

NUTS
EGGS
NIGHTSHADES
FODMAPS
SEAFOOD

1 avocado
1/4 cup grated cucumber
1 small clove garlic, grated
juice of 1 lemon

2 tablespoons extra-virgin olive oil
sea salt and black pepper to taste
1 teaspoon minced fresh dill

INGREDIENT TIP
*Check out page 224 for a list of recommended brands. ●

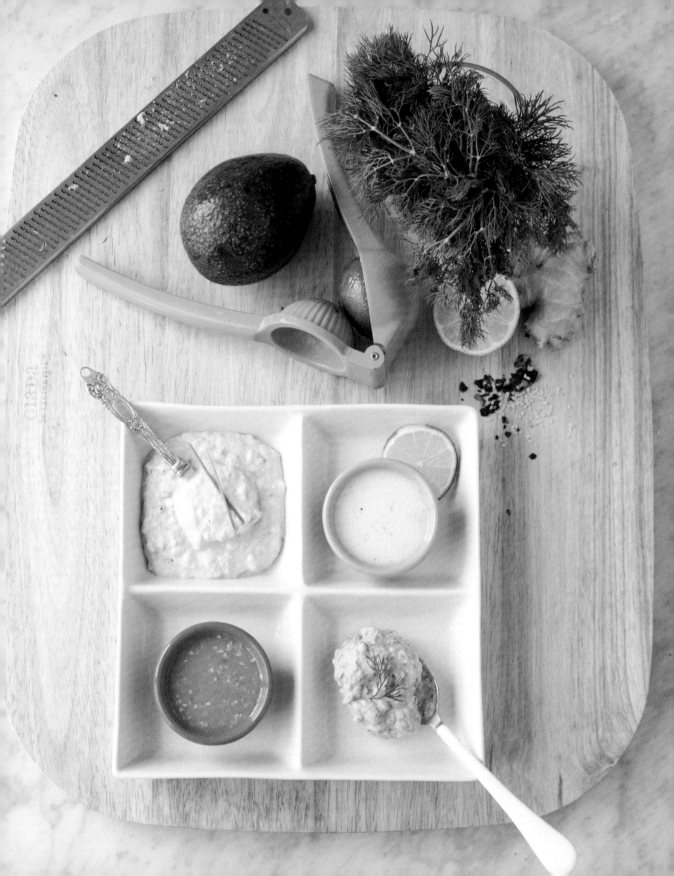

balsamic vinaigrette dressing

PREP TIME **5 MINS** • SERVINGS **8** • YIELD **1 CUP**

NUTS

EGGS

NIGHTSHADES

FODMAPS

SEAFOOD

1/3 cup balsamic vinegar

2/3 cup extra-virgin olive oil

1 teaspoon gluten-free Dijon mustard

1/2 teaspoon minced shallot or garlic

sea salt and black pepper to taste

1/2 teaspoon dried oregano or basil (optional)

Combine all the ingredients in a resealable glass jar and shake well to combine.

Label and store in the refrigerator for up to a month.

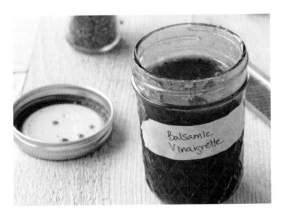

lemon-herb dressing

PREP TIME **5 MINS** • SERVINGS **8** • YIELD **1 CUP**

NUTS

EGGS

NIGHTSHADES

FODMAPS

SEAFOOD

1/3 cup fresh lemon juice

2/3 cup extra-virgin olive oil

1 teaspoon gluten-free Dijon mustard

1/2 teaspoon minced shallot

sea salt and black pepper to taste

1/2 teaspoon minced fresh cilantro or basil (optional)

Combine all the ingredients in a resealable glass jar and shake well to combine.

Label and store in the refrigerator for up to a month.

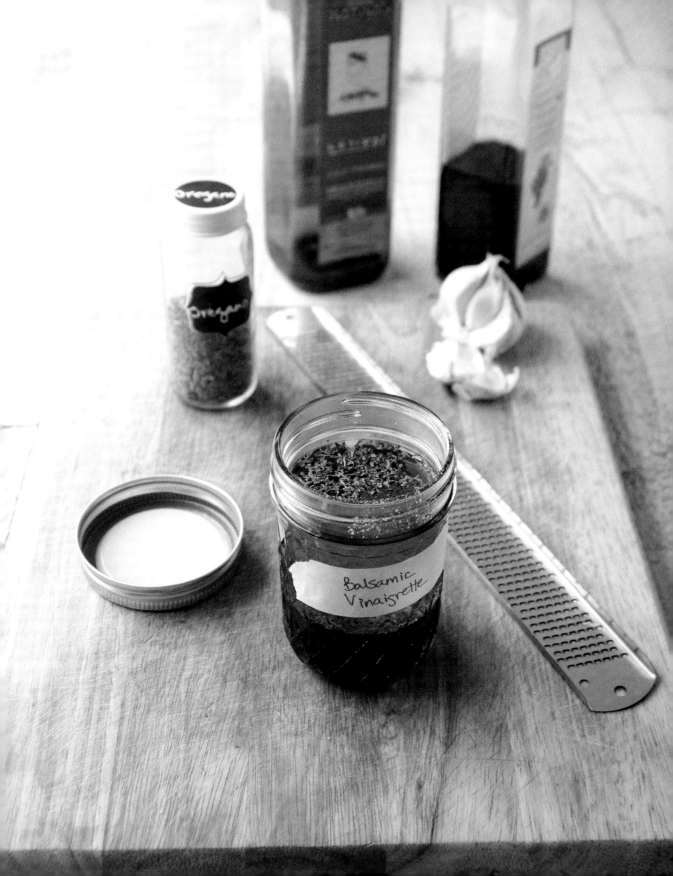

figuring out **your carb count**

your 21DSD plate may not look like your friend's—heads up!

SUFFICIENT CARBOHYDRATE INTAKE FROM GOOD CARBS!	GENERAL LIFESTYLE FACTORS: ACTIVITY & STRESS LEVELS
VERY LOW CARB*: **0–30G/DAY**	An inactive person or insulin-resistant person seeking to make drastic changes to their sugar metabolism; someone interested in a ketogenic diet approach; not recommended or necessary for most people seeking general, optimal health.
LOW CARB: **30–75G/DAY**	Not very active or participating in intense cardiovascular activity that lasts *fewer* than twenty minutes per day; also suitable for most weight-lifting and strength-training individuals; someone interested in a ketogenic diet approach (up to ~50g of carbs); **this is a healthy range for many people.**
MODERATE CARB: **75–150G/DAY**	Moderately active or completing intense cardiovascular activity that lasts between twenty and sixty minutes per day; a generally active job or lifestyle; a moderately stressful lifestyle; **this is a healthy range for many people.**
HIGHER CARB: **150G+/DAY** **(UP TO AROUND 300G)**	Participating intense cardiovascular activity that lasts more than sixty minutes per day; a very active job with consistent movement; a very stressful lifestyle that is mentally and physically demanding; **this is a healthy range for people who are very active or have very stressful lives.**

A prolonged very-low-carb approach is not recommended for most people, as you may miss out on some of the beneficial micronutrients available in carbohydrate-rich foods. While nose-to-tail animal food consumption that includes all organ meats would circumvent this issue, most people are not eating animals in this fashion today. Good carbs are also important for proper digestive function, as carbohydrates aid in balancing healthy gut flora (bacterial balance).

starchy **carbohydrate vegetables**

additional carb sources for those who are following the Energy modifications for all levels of the 21DSD program

ITEM NAME	CARBS PER 100G	FIBER PER 100G	CARBS PER 1 CUP	OTHER NOTABLE NUTRIENTS
cassava (raw)	38g	2g	78g	Vitamin C, Thiamin, Folate, Potassium, Manganese
taro root	35g	5g	46g, sliced	B6, Vitamin E, Potassium, Manganese
plantain	31g	2g	62g, mashed	Vitamin A (beta carotene), Vitamin C, B6, Magnesium, Potassium
yam	27g	4g	37g, cubed	Vitamin C, Vitamin B6, Manganese, Potassium
white potato	22g	1g	27g, peeled	trace Vitamin C
sweet potato	21g	3g	58g, mashed	Vitamin A (beta carotene), Vitamin C, B6, Potassium, Manganese, Magnesium, Iron, Vitamin E
parsnips	17g	4g	27g, sliced	Vitamin C, Manganese
lotus root	16g	3g	19g, sliced	Vitamin C, B6, Potassium, Copper, Manganese
winter squash	15g	4g	30g, cubed	Vitamin C, Thiamin, B6
onion	10g	1g	21g, chopped	Vitamin C, Potassium
beets	10g	2g	17g, sliced	Folate, Manganese
butternut squash	10g	-	22g	Vitamin A (beta carotene), Vitamin C

15 egg-free breakfast ideas

if you can't eat eggs or simply want a change of pace
for breakfasts, here are some combinations to try

1. Almond or Coconut Milk Smoothie (pages 92-93)

2. Mustard-Glazed Chicken Thighs (page 114), green vegetable

3. Green Apple Breakfast Sausage (page 94), green vegetable

4. Ground beef cooked with curry spice & cinnamon, butternut squash

5. Bacon-wrapped chicken thighs

6. Wild canned salmon with chopped avocado, olives, and lemon juice

7. Ground beef cooked with chopped bacon (cook with sea salt, black pepper, garlic powder, onion powder, and cinnamon) and spaghetti squash

8. Baked acorn squash with coconut butter and cinnamon, bacon or breakfast sausage

9. Rosemary Salmon with Cabbage (page 96)

10. Baked chicken thighs with curry powder and cinnamon, green apple, Swiss chard

11. Greek-style Meatballs (page 129) with Creamy Herb Mashed Cauliflower (page 178)

12. Smoked salmon nori (seaweed) hand roll with avocado, cucumber, and chives

13. Root Veggie Hash (page 95) with breakfast sausage

14. Baked chicken with rosemary, sea salt, and black pepper; sliced carrots with cinnamon sautéed in coconut oil

15. Turkey & bacon club salad: chopped romaine topped with sliced turkey breast, cooked bacon, tomatoes, and avocado

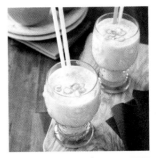
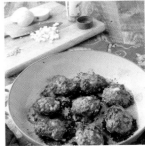
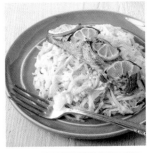
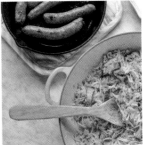

pinterest.com/21daysugardetox/autoimmune-breakfast/

For more ideas and inspiration, check out our Pinterest boards for autoimmune-friendly 21DSD breakfasts, all of which are grain, legume, dairy, egg, nightshade, nut, and seed tree

websites & blogs

these sites are maintained by recipe bloggers and a variety of people who have completed The 21DSD

RECIPE BLOGS

Against All Grain // **againstallgrain.com**
Chowstalker // **stalkerville.net**
Civilized Caveman Cooking Creations // **civilizedcavemancooking.com**
Fast Paleo // **fastpaleo.com**
The Food Lover's Primal Palate // **primalpalate.com**
Grass Fed Girl // **grassfedgirl.com**
The Paleo Mom // **thepaleomom.com**
Paleo Parents // **paleoparents.com**
The Paleo Pot // **paleopot.com**
The Paleo Professional // **thepaleoprofessional.blogspot.com**
PaleOMG // **paleomg.com**
TGIPaleo // **tgipaleo.com**
The Urban Poser // **theurbanposer.com**
Zenbelly Blog // **zenbellycatering.com**

21DSD EXPERIENCES

Babble + bloom // **babbleandbloom.com**
Butterflies, peace, paleo // **butterfliespeacepaleo.blogspot.com**
ExSoyCise // **exsoycise.com**
Fire Wifey // **firewifey.com**
Fresh 4 Five // **fresh4five.com**
Funky's Evolution // **funkysevolution.blogspot.com**
Half Indian Cook // **halfindiancook.com**
Healthy Mom on the Run // **healthymomontherun.com**
Naturally Homemade // **naturallyhomemade.blogspot.com**
Oh me of little faith // **ohmeoflittlefaith.com**
Paleo Foodie Kitchen // **paleofoodiekitchen.com**
Popular Paleo // **popularpaleo.com**
Purplekat's Kitchen // **purplekatskitchen.blogspot.com**
South Beach Primal // **southbeachprimal.com**
The Paleo Prize // **thepaleoprize.com**
The Rudd Manor Kitchen // **kristenrudd.com**

balancedbites.com/21DSD
All of these websites and blogs are linked to on the book resources page on my website for easy access anytime.

recommended **products & brands**

for your 21DSD and beyond, listed
in alphabetical order within each category

FRESH**PRODUCTS**

APPLEGATE FARMS MEATS
Most grocery stores
Deli meats, bacon

BUBBIES SAUERKRAUT
Most grocery stores
All flavors approved; when in doubt,
check ingredients

FAB FERMENTS
Online: fabferments.com

G.T.'S SYNERGY
Whole Foods Market, most grocery stores
Kombucha: various flavors

PETE'S PALEO
Online: petespaleo.com
21DSD-approved meals, bacon

REAL PICKLES
*Whole Foods Market, local organic
grocers/co-ops*

TESSEMAE'S ALL NATURAL
*Online: tessemaes.com; Whole Foods
Market*
Dressing/marinade/dip: Balsamic,
Cracked Pepper, Hot Sauce/Wing
Sauce (mild, medium, hot), Oil-
Free Italian, Lemon Chesapeake,
Lemon Garlic, Lemonette, Red Wine
Vinaigrette, Zesty Ranch
Excludes Soy Ginger & Matty's BBQ
(I recommend adding Kasandrinos
Extra Virgin Olive Oil to the oil-free
varieties if you purchase those)

WHOLLY GUACAMOLE
*Online: eatwholly.com; Whole Foods
Market, Trader Joe's (as store brand),
Costco, local organic grocers/co-ops*

WILDBRINE
*Whole Foods Market, local organic
grocers/co-ops*
Sauerkraut: various flavors

21DSD **JERKY**

PALEO JERKY
Online: huntedandgathered.com.au
Note: The sugar content is negligible,
so this jerky is okay for The 21DSD.

SOPHIA'S SURVIVAL FOOD
Online: grassfedjerkychews.com
Beef jerky: Mild and Spicy
*Excludes Chipotle Raisin flavor—which
is fantastic for after your 21DSD!*

STEVE'S ORIGINAL
Online: stevespaleogoods.com
Just Jerky & PaleoStix varieties
*Excludes Berky, Dried Fruit, PaleoKits,
and PaleoKrunch*

US WELLNESS MEATS
Online: bit.ly/USWMBB
Jerky, Pemmican
Excludes Honey & Cherry flavor

FATS&**OILS**

ARTISANA & NUTIVA BRANDS
*Online: artisana.com, Amazon.com; local
grocers*
Coconut oil

FATWORKS
Online: fatworksfoods.com
Duck fat, lard, and tallow

KASANDRINOS OLIVE OIL
Online: kasandrinos.com

KERRYGOLD BUTTER
*Trader Joe's, Costco, Whole Foods
Market, local grocers*

PURE INDIAN FOODS GHEE
*Online: pureindianfoods.com,
Amazon.com; local grocers*

SMJÖR BUTTER
Grocery stores

TROPICAL TRADITIONS
See also: Nuts & Baking Items
Online: tropicaltraditions.com
Coconut oil (I recommend Green Label
for the best taste)

WILDERNESS FAMILY NATURALS
Online: wildernessfamilynaturals.com
Organic coconut oils, natural red palm
oil, sesame seed oil, olive oil, Mary's
Sauté Oil named after Mary Enig,
author of *Know Your Fats* (blend of
virgin coconut oil, extra-virgin olive oil,
and unrefined sesame seed oil)

SAUCES&**DRESSINGS**
See also: Fresh Products

ANNIE'S & EDEN FOODS
*Online: Amazon.com; Whole Foods
Market, local grocers*
Gluten-free mustards

ARIZONA GUNSLINGER
*Online: azgunslinger.com; selected
retailers*
Organic harvest gluten-free hot sauces

BIONATURAE
*Online: tropicaltraditions.com;
Whole Foods Market*
Balsamic vinegar

BRAGG'S
Local grocers
Organic apple cider vinegar

COCONUT SECRET
*Online: coconutsecret.com, Amazon.
com; Whole Foods Market, local organic
grocers/co-ops*
Coconut aminos, coconut vinegar

FRANKS REDHOT
*Online: franksredhot.com, Amazon.com;
major grocery stores*

RED BOAT FISH SAUCE
*Online: redboatfishsauce.com; Whole
Foods Market, local grocers*

If specific products aren't listed, then you will likely find that all of their products are 21DSD-friendly. But please check ingredients on all packages, and take note of your level and modification guides as well.

For web links to all of these products & more, visit: balancedbites.com/21DSD

COCONUT, NUTS
BUTTERS&FLOURS

ARTISANA & NUTIVA BRANDS
Online: artisana.com, Amazon.com; local organic grocers/co-ops
Almond butter (roasted or raw), coconut butter, coconut manna—sold in jars and handy travel-sized packets.
Excludes cashew, walnut, pecan, and macadamia butters (all are blended with cashews), & Cacao Bliss—which are fantastic for after your 21DSD!

BARNEY BUTTER
Online: barneybutter.com, Amazon.com
Barney Bare only
Excludes smooth, crunchy, and squeeze packs (at this time, the Barney Bare is not available in squeeze packs)

BOB'S RED MILL
Online: bobsredmill.com, Amazon.com; major grocery stores
Almond, coconut, hazelnut meal/flours

HONEYVILLE
Online: honeyville.com
Blanched almond meal/flour

JUSTIN'S NUT BUTTER
Online: justins.com, Amazon.com; local grocers
Original only—sold in jars and handy travel-sized packets
Excludes honey, maple, chocolate, and vanilla almond butters, all peanut butters, and chocolate hazelnut butter

MARANATHA
Online: maranathafoods.com, Amazon.com; Whole Foods Market, organic grocers
Almond butters, sunflower seed butter, sesame tahini

ONCE AGAIN NUT BUTTERS
Online: onceagainnutbutter.com; Whole Foods Market
Almond butter, tahini

PALEO MEENUT BUTTER
Online: meeeatpaleo.com

SUNBUTTER (NUT-FREE)
Online: sunbutter.com, Amazon.com; grocery stores
Only the Organic, unsweetened variety

THAI KITCHEN
Online: Amazon.com; grocery stores
Full-fat coconut milk, canned

TRADER JOE'S
traderjoes.com for locations
sunflower seed butter (unsweetened—read ingredients), almond butter

TROPICAL TRADITIONS
Online: tropicaltraditions.com
Shredded coconut, coconut chips, coconut flour, coconut cream concentrate

WHOLE FOODS STORE BRAND
wholefoodsmarket.com for locations
Full-fat coconut milk

WILDERNESS FAMILY NATURALS
Online: wildernessfamilynaturals.com
Coconut, coconut flour, coconut cream concentrate, almonds, crispy almonds, almond butter

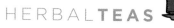

HERBAL TEAS

TRADITIONAL MEDICINALS
Online: Amazon.com; Whole Foods Market, local organic grocers/co-ops
All herbal tea varieties

BAKING ITEMS

IF YOU CARE, PAPER CHEF BRANDS
Online: Amazon.com; Whole Foods Market, local organic grocers/co-ops
Unbleached parchment paper muffin liners

REAL SALT
Online: realsalt.com, Amazon.com; grocery stores nationwide
Various unrefined salts

TROPICAL TRADITIONS
See also: Fats & Oils and Nuts
Online: tropicaltraditions.com
Cocoa powder, shredded coconut

WILDERNESS FAMILY NATURALS
Online: wildernessfamilynaturals.com
Organic raw cocoa powder, organic herbs & spices, natural unrefined salts

PANTRY ITEMS

BEAR & WOLF CANNED
Online: Amazon.com; Costco
Wild-caught salmon

BIONATURAE, JOVIAL, & POMI BRANDS
Online: tropicaltraditions.com; Whole Foods Market, local organic grocers/co-ops
Tomato products, strained tomatoes, chopped tomatoes

EMERALD COVE & EDEN FOODS
Grocery stores, Asian markets
Nori (dried seaweed paper)

IMPROVE'EAT
Online: improveat.com
Wraps

MEDITERRANEAN ORGANIC
Online: Amazon; local grocers
Olives, other grocery items—read labels

MOUNTAIN ROSE HERBS
Online: mountainroseherbs.com
Herbs & spices

SEASNAX
Online: seasnax.com; grocery stores

WILD PLANET
Online: Amazon.com; grocery stores
Canned sardines, wild-caught salmon

Introduction

Ervin, R. Bethene, and Cynthia L. Ogden. *Consumption of Added Sugars Among U.S. Adults*, 2005–2010, NCHS Data Brief no. 122. Hyattsville, MD: National Center for Health Statistics, 2013.

Bowman, Shanthy A., James E. Friday, and Alanna J. Moshfegh. *MyPyramid Equivalents Database, 2.0 for USDA Survey Foods, 2003-2004*. Beltsville, MD: U.S. Department of Agriculture, 2008. http://www.ars.usda.gov/ba/bhnrc/fsrg/.

Calton, Jayson, and Mira Calton. *Rich Food Poor Food*. Malibu, CA: Primal Nutrition, Inc., 2013.

Mercola, Joseph. Sweet Deception: *Why Splenda, NutraSweet, and the FDA May Be Hazardous to Your Health*. Nashville, TN: Thomas Nelson, 2006.

Yang, Qing. "Gain Weight by 'Going Diet'? Artificial Sweeteners and the Neurobiology of Sugar Cravings." *Yale Journal of Biology and Medicine* 83, no. 2 (2010): 101-108.

The Science of Sugar – Simplified

www.nutritiondata.com

Kulp, Karel, and Joseph G. Ponte. *Handbook of Cereal Technology*. New York: Marcel Dekker, 2000.

Kjær, Michael, Michael Krogsgaard, Peter Magnusson, Lars Engebretsen, Harald Roos, Timo Takala, and Savio L-Y Woo. *Textbook of Sports Medicine: Basic Science and Clinical Aspects of Sports Injury and Physical Activity*. Malden, MA: Blackwell Science, Ltd., 2003.

Avena, Nicole M., P. Rada, and B. G. Hoebel. "Evidence for Sugar Addiction: Behavioral and Neurochemical Effects of Intermittent, Excessive Sugar Intake." *Neuroscience and Biobehavioral Reviews* 32, no. 1 (2008): 20-39.

Ferland, Annie, Patrice Bassard, and Paul Poirier. "Is Aspartame Really Safer in Reducing the Risk of Hypoglycemia During Exercise in Patients with Type 2 Diabetes?" *Diabetes Care* 30, no. 7 (2007): E59.

Supplements

Murray, Michael T. *Encyclopedia of Nutritional Supplements: The Essential Guide for Improving Your Health Naturally*. Roseville, CA: Prima Publishing, 1996.

Segala, Melanie. *The Life Extension Foundation's Disease Prevention and Treatment: Scientific Protocols That Integrate Mainstream and Alternative Medicine*. Hollywood, FL: Life Extension Media, 2003.

FAQs

Truss, C. Orian. "Restoration of Immunologic Competence to Candida Albicans." *Orthomolecular Psychiatry* 9, no. 4 (1980): 287-301.

balancedbites.com/21DSD

For hyperlinks to each of these sources, please visit the book resources web page.

recipe **index**

MAIN **DISHES**

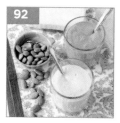
92
almond milk
smoothies

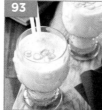
93
coconut milk
smoothies

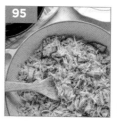
94
green apple
breakfast sausage

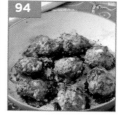
95
bacon & root
veggie hash

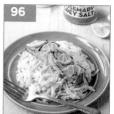
96
rosemary salmon
with cabbage

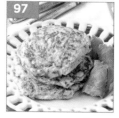
97
veggie pancakes

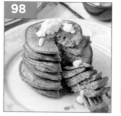
98
pumpkin pancakes
with vanilla bean
coconut butter

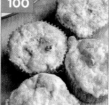
100
buffalo chicken
egg muffins

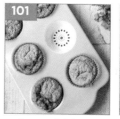
101
broccoli & herb
egg muffins

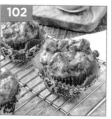
102
apple streusel
egg muffins

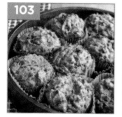
103
carrot pumpkin
spice muffins

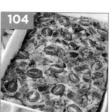
104
tomato-basil quiche
with bacon &
spinach

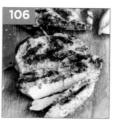
106
perfectly grilled
chicken breast

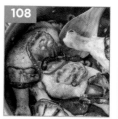
108
chicken with tri-color
peppers

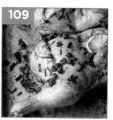
109
lemon chicken with
capers & chives

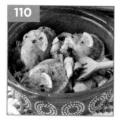
110
chicken with
artichokes & olives

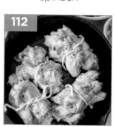
112
parsnip & bacon
stuffed chicken
roll-ups

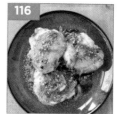
114
mustard-glazed
chicken thighs

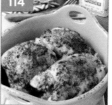
116
hot & sweet ginger-
garlic chicken

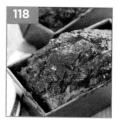
118
mini mexi-
meatloaves

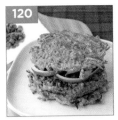
120

jalapeño bacon
burgers

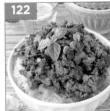
122

spaghetti squash
bolognese

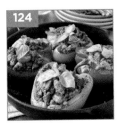
124

italian-style stuffed
bell peppers

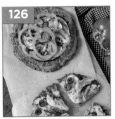
126

meatza two-ways

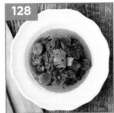
128

balsamic-braised
beef

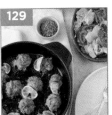
129

greek-style
meatballs & salad

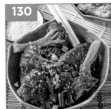
130

ginger-garlic
beef & broccoli

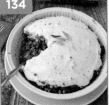
132

crunchy curried
beef lettuce cups

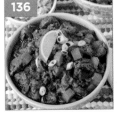
134

shepherd's pie

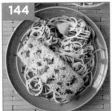
136

stovetop lamb
& chorizo chili

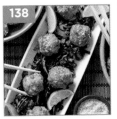
138

asian-style meatballs

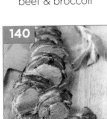
140

double pork
tenderloin

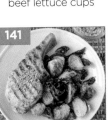
141

cinnamon grilled
pork chops

142

seafood & chorizo
paella

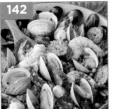
144

spicy sesame-lime
salmon

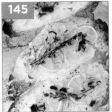
145

lemon sole with
almonds & thyme

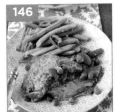
146

broiled salmon
with caper & olive
tapenade

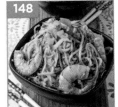
148

shrimp pad thai

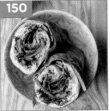
150

rainbow collard
wraps with herb
almond "cheese"
spread

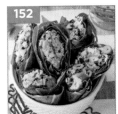
152

tuna salad wraps

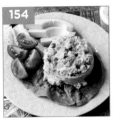
154

salmon salad with
capers & tomato

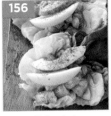
156

buffalo shrimp
lettuce cups

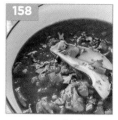
158

smoky chicken
tortilla-less soup

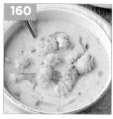
160

roasted cauliflower
soup

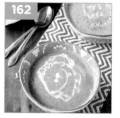
162

simple spinach &
garlic soup

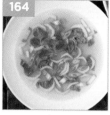
164

no-miso soup

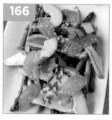
166

seared tuna,
grapefruit, &
asparagus salad

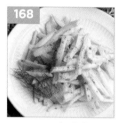
168

green apple & fennel
salad

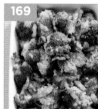
169

broccoli & bacon
salad with creamy
balsamic dressing

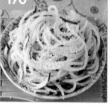
170

cucumber cold
noodle salad

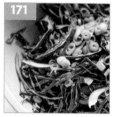
171

fresh cabbage & bok
choy slaw

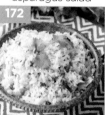
172

basic cilantro
cauli-rice

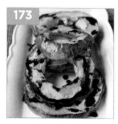
173

balsamic winter
squash rings

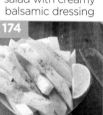
174

jicama fresh "fries"

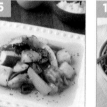
175

greek tomato &
cucumber salad

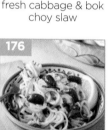
176

lemon & garlic
noodles with olives

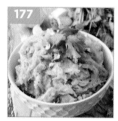
177

pesto spaghetti
squash

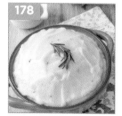
178

creamy herb mashed
cauliflower

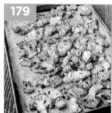
179

cocoa-chili roasted
cauliflower

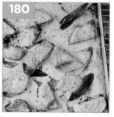
180

golden beets with
crispy herbs

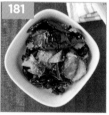
181

crumb-topped
brussels sprouts

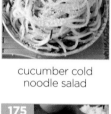

SNACKS

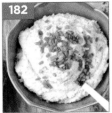
182
herb almond
"cheese" spread

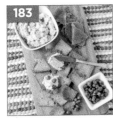
183
herb crackers

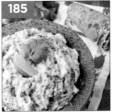
184
simple beef jerky

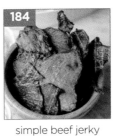
185
basic 4 guacamole

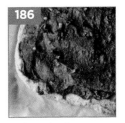
186
tomato & green
onion faux-caccia

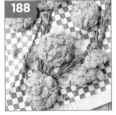
188
savory herb drop
biscuits

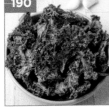
190
baked kale chips

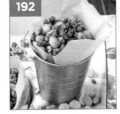
192
cinnilla nut mix

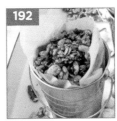
192
spicy thai nut mix

NOT-SWEET **TREATS**

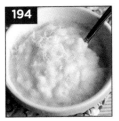
194
tart & creamy
applesauce

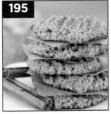
195
not-sweet cinnamon
cookies

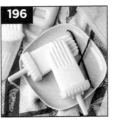
196
vanilla bean coconut
freezer pops

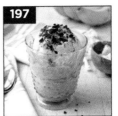
197
banana coconut
ice cream

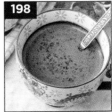
198
bittersweet hot
cocoa

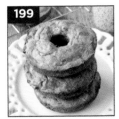
199
apple cinnamon
donuts

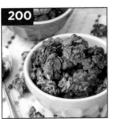
200
grain-free
banola

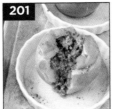
201
nutty baked apples

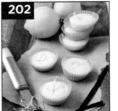
202
lemon vanilla
meltaways

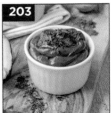
203
moo-less chocolate
mousse

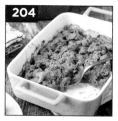
granny smith apple crumble

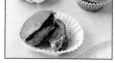
almond butter cups

KITCHEN **BASICS**

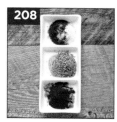
spice blends

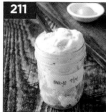
clarified butter & ghee

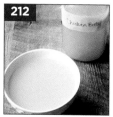
healthy homemade mayonnaise

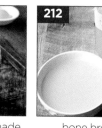
bone broth

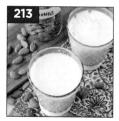
almond milk & meal

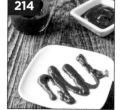
sweetener-free ketchup

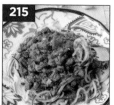
simple marinara

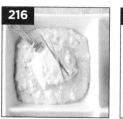
avo-goddess sauce

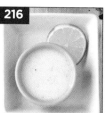
creamy ginger lime dressing

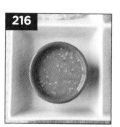
spicy sesame ginger dressing

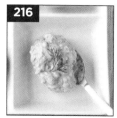
avo-ziki sauce

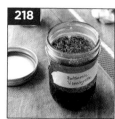
balsamic vinaigrette dressing

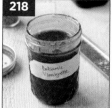
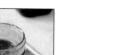
lemon-herb dressing

index

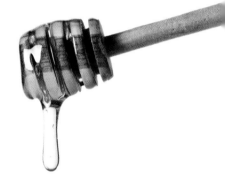

ingredient **index**

nutrition facts for all recipes can be found online at balancedbites.com/21DSD

my thanks

"Feeling gratitude and not expressing it is like wrapping a present and not giving it." —William Arthur Ward

Mom & Dad

There is no way I could ever thank anyone before my parents. You both have always supported me and my passions unconditionally. Thanks for being there for trips to the airport, for grocery-store runs, and to eat (and critique) the extra food from recipe development for this book! I'm sure that was the toughest part, right?

Grandma

Though I can't promise you great-grandchildren, I am offering up another book "grandbaby"! I am so excited to share the fruits of my labor with you once again so that you can see what your lineage is leaving behind as a mark on this world.

Scott

There aren't enough words to express how grateful I am for the calm and balance you have brought to my life over the last year. I know I made it through this book with more sanity than I would have on my own because you were there for me—my rock. I'm so lucky that you are in my life. You're my favorite.

My Brazen family

Link, Big J, C, Alex, Rebecca, Cass, Britt, Shelly, Greco, Big & Little V, Jecks... and *everyone* at Brazen Athletics: You guys have no idea how much I've appreciated having my Brazen family to come home to, to count on, to talk about life and love with, and to lift heavy things with over this last year. The amount of positive energy and inspiration that comes from Brazen is unmatched. I've trained in many, many gyms, but I call Brazen my home—it is way more than a gym—and I'm honored to do so. You are all LIMITLESS. I love you.

Charissa

You've taken charge of growing the reach of The 21DSD and have supported everyone on the program like a boss! I could not have taken things to this level if you hadn't been so dedicated. Thanks for running the show behind the scenes over the years, and for supporting our entire team with vigor and excitement. I'm certain I wouldn't have had the strength to put this program into a printed book if you hadn't been there to help out every step of the way.

Brooke, Rebekah, Shannon, Eric, Ellen, Trecia, April, and all of the 21DSD moderators

The amount of time you all spend helping others who are participating in The 21DSD is simply insane. I can't ever thank you enough for that, and I look forward to seeing how your expertise will continue to support those who embark on this sugar-free journey with us.

All of the bloggers who have embraced this program

Some of you have completed it and helped share it through your experiences, while others of you have created 21DSD-friendly recipes—and many of you have done both! In every case, your support for my work and for the program that is helping tens of thousands of people is just amazing. I appreciate every minute and every hour that you've spent putting your photos and posts together, as I know how much time they take.

Pam

Thanks for talking me off the ledge when I felt like this book could never say everything I ever wanted to tell people about sugar and carbs. Realizing that this book is meant to help them through just three weeks, and not an entire lifetime, put me at ease to get the work wrapped up without completely going insane.

Erich, Michele, and everyone on the Victory Belt team

Once again you have all supported me and my crazy book-creation process in a way that I'm certain no other publishing company would do. Through the meltdowns and the circular content development, you guys have pushed me through the tough spots and cheered me on the entire time. I'm happy to be a part of the family.

Everyone who has already completed The 21DSD

Thank you for being engaged, inquisitive, motivated, and determined to crush this program with all your might! The tens of thousands of you who have come before the many more tens of thousands who will eventually find this book, well, you've paved the way. It was through your experiences that I was able to craft much of the richer content in this book. Keep sharing your words of wisdom with one another in the online communities, as you are the ones to pass the torch to others who seek to improve their health as you did.

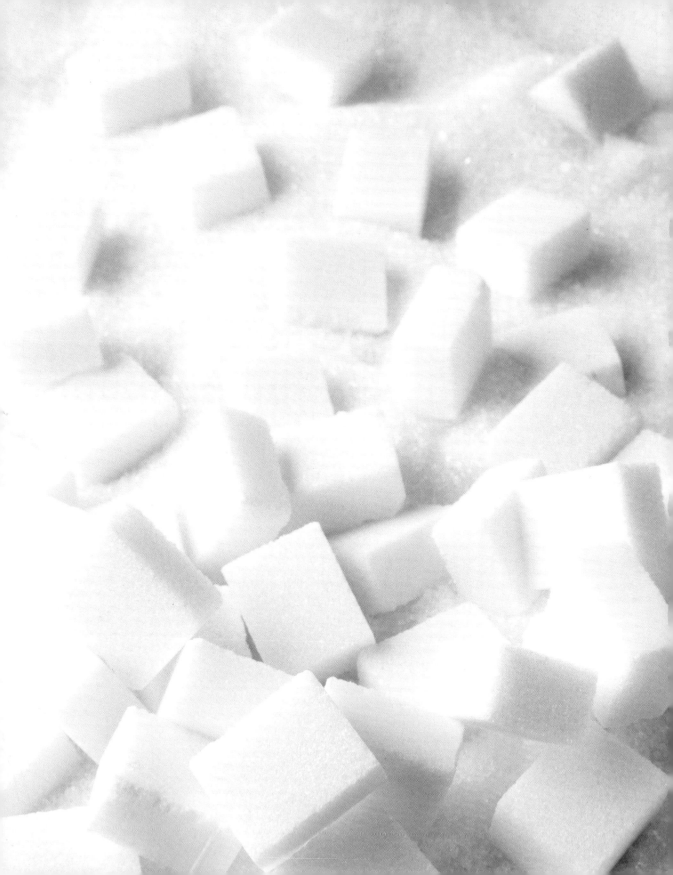